Encountering
the Plague

BCMCR
New Directions in Media and Cultural Research

Series editors: Oliver Carter, Kirsten Forkert, Nicholas Gebhardt, and Dima Saber.
Print ISSN: 2752-4515 | **Online ISSN:** 2752-4523

The Birmingham Centre for Media and Cultural Research's 'New Directions' book series aims to advance research and teaching in the broad range of media and cultural studies and to serve as the focal point for a community of scholars who are committed to critical inquiry and collaborative practice. Books in the series engage with developments in the field, showing how new theoretical approaches have impacted on research within both media and cultural studies and other related disciplines. Each volume will focus on a specific theme or issue, as well as exploring broader processes of social and cultural transformation. The series is committed to producing distinctive titles that challenge traditional disciplinary boundaries and question existing paradigms, including innovative scholarship in areas such as the creative industries; media history, heritage and archives; games studies; gender and sexuality; screen cultures; jazz and popular music studies; media and conflict; song-writing studies; and critical theory. The editors are also keen to encourage authors to experiment with non-standard approaches to academic writing.

In this series:

Under the Counter: Britain's Trade in Hardcore Pornographic 8mm Films, by Oliver Carter (2023)
Media Materialities: Form, Format, and Ephemeral Meaning, edited by Iain Taylor and Oliver Carter (2023)
Encountering the Plague: Humanities takes on the Pandemic, edited by Wojciech Sowa, Tony Whyton (2024)

Encountering the Plague

Humanities Takes on the Pandemic

EDITED BY

Wojciech Sowa and Tony Whyton

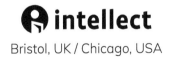

Bristol, UK / Chicago, USA

First published in the UK in 2024 by
Intellect, The Mill, Parnall Road, Fishponds, Bristol, BS16 3JG, UK

First published in the USA in 2024 by
Intellect, The University of Chicago Press, 1427 E. 60th Street,
Chicago, IL 60637, USA

The publication of this book was made possible through the generous support of the Humanities in the European Research Area (HERA).

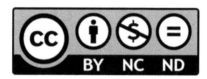

https://creativecommons.org/licenses/by-nc-nd/4.0/
Some rights reserved. Without limiting the rights under copyright reserved above, any part of this book may be reproduced, stored in or introduced into a retrieval system, or transmitted, in any form or by any means (electronic, mechanical, photocopying, recording or otherwise).

A catalogue record for this book is available from the British Library.

Copy editor: MPS Limited
Cover designer: Tanya Montefusco
Cover image: Gwengoat
Stock illustration ID:145031089
Production manager: Julie Willis (Westchester Publishing Services UK)
Typesetter: MPS Limited

Hardback ISBN 978-1-78938-986-9
Paperback ISBN 978-1-78938-987-6
ePDF ISBN 978-1-78938-989-0
ePUB ISBN 978-1-78938-988-3

To find out about all our publications, please visit our website. There you can subscribe to our e-newsletter, browse or download our current catalogue and buy any titles that are in print.

www.intellectbooks.com

This is a peer-reviewed publication.

Contents

List of Figures	vii
Acknowledgements	ix

INTRODUCTION	1
1. Encountering the Plague *Wojciech Sowa and Tony Whyton*	3

RITUALS AND RITES, RIGHTS AND BEHAVIOURS	15
2. Heritage, Escapism and Anxiety: Visits to Corfe Castle during the COVID-19 Pandemic *Joanna Sofaer*	17
3. Ritualization of 'Distance' in Christian Liturgy During the Plague *Piotr Roszak and Piotr Paweł Orłowski*	38
4. Protesting in Defence of Human Rights in the Time of Pandemic: Freedom of Assembly and COVID-19 *Grażyna Baranowska and Aleksandra Gliszczyńska-Grabias*	54

PLAGUE IN HISTORY	69
5. Recounting the Plague in Sixteenth and Seventeenth-Century London *Charles Giry-Deloison*	71
6. Representation of the Plague in Ancient Greek and Byzantine Texts and Responses to the COVID-19 Pandemic *Florian Steger*	93

7. 'Let every man drinke in his own cup, and let none trust the breath   107
of his brother': Encountering Plague in Early Modern Port Cities
James Brown and Gabrielle Robilliard

COVID-19: TEXTS AND DISCOURSE   125

8. Coronavirus in Times of the Late Internet: Compulsive Visualization   127
and a Data-Hungry Society
Agnieszka Jelewska
9. How Language Conceptualized the Pandemic   147
Małgorzata Majewska
10. Pandemic Discourse: From Intimidation to Social Distancing   157
Rūta Petrauskaitė and Darius Amilevičius

CREATIVE RESPONSES TO PLAGUE   179

11. Nights of Crises and Resistance: (En)countering the Politics of   181
Disease and Death in *Bacurau* (2019)
Sara Brandellero
12. A Pandemic Crisis Seen from the Screen: A Reflection on Pandemic   193
Imagination
Anna Nacher, Søren Bro Pold and Scott Rettberg
13. Repetition and Revision: *The Plague*, 'St James' and the Humanities   214
in Times of Crisis
Tony Whyton

CONCLUSION   225

14. The Power of the Humanities   227
Wojciech Sowa

List of Contributors   233
Index   241

Figures

1.1: A Hittite cuneiform tablet. Courtesy of hethiter.net/: fotarch N03613. — 3
2.1: Samuel Hieronymus Grimm (1733–94) Corfe Castle. Ink wash on paper (1790). British Library f.131. — 17
2.2: Corfe Castle in 2020. Photo: J. Sofaer. — 25
3.1: The streaming of a holy mass during the COVID-19 pandemic. Courtesy of https://media.defense.gov/ ⓢ. — 38
4.1: Picture of protesters with facemasks taking part in mass protests against the abortion judgement in Poland in October 2020, Łukasz Cynalewski, Gazeta Wyborcza. — 54
5.1: Nathaniel HODGES, *Loimologia: or, an Historical Account of the Plague in London in 1665* […], London, printed for E. Bell and J. Osborn, 1721, 3rd ed., p. 7. Paris: Bibliothèque nationale de France, 8-TD53-190. — 71
6.1: Unknown artist (possibly Guillaume Spicre), circa 1446. *Trionfo della Morte* (*Triumph of Death*). Originally in Palazzo Sclafani, now in Palermo's Regional Gallery, Palazzo Abatellis. — 93
7.1: Cruikshank, George, *A cart for transporting the dead in London during the great plague* (1833), Watercolour painting. 18.5 × 14 cm. The Wellcome Collection. Courtesy of the Wellcome Collection ⓢ. — 107
8.1: COVID-19 Dashboard by the Center for Systems Science and Engineering (CSSE) at Johns Hopkins University, screenshot from 28 May 2021. — 127
8.2: Visualizing the virus, curated clusters, screenshot from 10 May 2022. — 140

9.1:	Cartoon representing what our mind does with something new for which we lack the language. Courtesy of Maciek Dziadyk.	147
9.2:	Cartoon representing how we tame difficult words through language. When something that scares us gets a name, we have the false sense that we can somehow control it. Courtesy of Maciek Dziadyk.	152
10.1:	Anon. *Intimidating headlines*. Black and white photograph. Courtesy of iStock.	157
10.2:	Anon. *Social distancing*. Black and white photograph. Courtesy of iStock.	159
10.3:	*A Wordle of Coronavirus* headlines from Lithuanian news portals. Image: Darius Amilevičius.	160
11.1:	Frame grab from *Bacurau*, 2019. Courtesy of Kleber Mendonça Filho, at Cinemascopio.	181
12.1:	Jörg Piringer: *Covid-19 genome* poem, screenshot from Piringer's 'Quarantine TV'. Courtesy of the artist.	193
12.2:	Ben Grosser: screenshot from *USA COVID-19 deaths visualized by the footprint of the 9/11 Memorial in NYC* (Instagram). Courtesy of the artist.	198
12.3:	Jody Zellen: screenshot from *Ghost City, Avenue S*. Courtesy of the artist.	201
12.4:	Screenshot from *Coronário* by Giselle Beiguelman. Courtesy of the artist.	202
12.5:	Screenshot from *The Endless Doomscroller* by Ben Grosser. Courtesy of the artist.	204
13.1:	Albert Camus' *The Plague* and Cab Calloway's 'St James Infirmary'. Photo: Tony Whyton.	214
14.1:	A screenshot from Annlin Chao's animation *Humanities Matter* (2020).	227

Acknowledgements

This book was funded by the HERA Joint Research Programme. The editors were supported by the 'Excellence Initiative – Research University' fund at the Jagiellonian University, Krakow (Sowa), and the Arts, Design and Media 'Faculty Research Investment Scheme', Birmingham City University (Whyton).

We would like to thank the Humanities in the European Research Area Joint Research Programme (JRP) Board for their support in putting this book project together. The HERA JRP has played a significant role in championing transnational humanities research for over 15 years now and this collection provides a useful snapshot of work linked to different humanities subjects and JRP themes. The HERA JRP Board is drawn from experts and research council representatives across 26 member countries; each member has endorsed this project and supported our commitment to Gold Open Access publishing.

Tim Mitchell, Professor Nicholas Gebhardt (BCU) and the team at Intellect deserve a particular note of gratitude for their continued enthusiasm and encouragement and for their critical appraisal of the initial proposal; we really valued your understanding and ability to ask important questions at an early stage of development. We would also like to thank Jory Debenham for her initial proof-reading and copy-editing work that ensured a consistency of approach across all contributions and disciplines and the anonymous peer reviewers who provided encouragement for the work we were undertaking.

We would also like to thank the contributors for their enthusiasm and commitment to this book project, and for their professionalism in delivering chapters and supporting materials on time. Each contributor has had a link to the HERA programme in some way, either through participation in transnational projects, working as a HERA Board member, or through engagement with HERA Conferences, workshops and events as an invited speaker. We thank you all for your contributions!

Wojciech Sowa and Tony Whyton

INTRODUCTION

1

Encountering the Plague

Wojciech Sowa and Tony Whyton

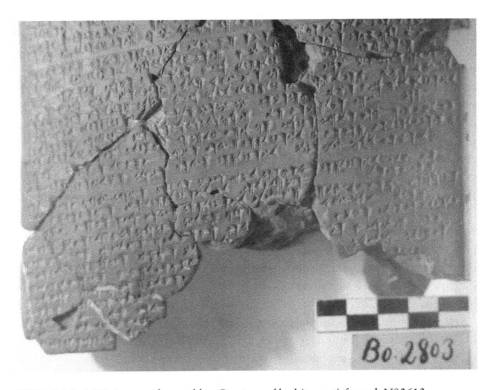

FIGURE 1.1: A Hittite cuneiform tablet. Courtesy of hethiter.net/: fotarch N03613.

Plague Prayers

Epidemics have been with us since long before the dawn of history. The crises caused by massive diseases form part of the basic experiences of mankind, as evidenced by the archaeological findings from ancient cultures such as Afanasievo, Corded Ware, Andronovo, Unetice or Sintashta. Within these contexts, the earliest traces of plague date to *c.*3000 BCE and stretch from Siberia to the areas of today's Estonia or Poland. Epidemics, mostly caused by the *Yersinia pestis* (namely plague), accompanied the rise of civilization and deeply affected the development of culture, society and the economies of ancient, mediaeval and modern societies.[1] As we all have seen recently, the COVID-19 crisis posed immense challenges not only to healthcare, medicine and science (such as the race for the vaccine), but also to society as a whole, and we are still being confronted with the political, economic, social and cultural effects of the newly emerged SARS-CoV-2 virus. COVID-19 demonstrated clearly that, despite decades of grand scientific and technological advancements, including medical breakthroughs, humans are still vulnerable and largely defenceless towards infectious diseases.

The impacts of epidemics and pandemics have long-lasting effects and affect the entire sphere of human activity, from individuals to communities. This situation is not new of course, and historical sources inform us about a whole range of issues connected with the spread of disease. Being aware of varied realities of the moment we are living in while looking to the past (e.g. contrasting modern times to the Mediaeval Black Death), we may compare various historical sources and try to observe a similar sequence of facts which seem to recur and testify, more or less, to repeated patterns of behaviours and responses of individuals and societies. One of the best examples of these historic testimonies is evidenced in documents from Ancient Anatolia. In the fourteenth century BCE, the Hittite Empire reached its peak under the reign of Suppiluliuma I. The empire dominated the entire area of Asia Minor and beyond, and became one of the biggest political players internationally alongside Assyria and Egypt. In this period, however, the Hittite Empire was devastated by an epidemic of tularemia, or 'rabbit fever'. This epidemic afflicted the Hittites for decades, killing the king and his son Arnuwanda II; the outbreak weakened the state and resulted in conflicts with its neighbours. By the times of the new king Mursilis (1321–1295 BCE), the lengthy plague had killed a large number of people, and the young leader was left with the difficult task of both investigating the reasons for the calamity and putting an end to the epidemic. The king started to cry to the gods for relief, and his plea has been preserved until today on a set of eight surviving cuneiform tablets that are specifically labelled 'Plague Prayers' (see Figure 1.1) from this period. Mursilis speaks on behalf of his people, and his distress at being unable to alleviate his nation's suffering is apparent:

INTRODUCTION

> O Storm-god of Hatti, my lord! [O gods], my lords! Mursili, your servant, has sent me saying: 'Go speak to the Storm-god of Hatti, my lord, and to the gods, my lords': What is this that you have done? You have allowed a plague into Hatti, so that Hatti has been very badly oppressed by the plague. People kept dying in the time of my father, in the time of my brother, and since I have become priest of the gods, they keep on dying in my time. For twenty years now people have been dying in Hatti. Will the plague never be removed from Hatti? I cannot control the worry of my heart, I can no longer control the anguish of my soul.
>
> (Singer 2002: 57–61)

Being presented in the form of prayers, the tablets invoke the gods through rituals that tie the objects to broader mythological practices. The inscriptions on these stones are ascribed to the highest king of the Hittites and the text suggests that divine wrath could be the cause of a horrific plague that is devastating the region. The 'Plague Prayers' stress the need for oracular consultation and look for divine intervention, moving beyond a desire for the simple understanding of medical causes of the epidemic towards the question of who is to blame for this extreme disruption to the workings of everyday life. Here, the tablets serve as both symbolic texts and as a chronicle of events, as they outline a twenty-year period of suffering. The inscription, translated as, 'to mankind, our wisdom has been lost and whatever we do right comes to nothing' gives us a sense that the chain of normal human life and its associated rituals are broken, which in turn has led to a disruption in moral codes and everyday relationships. The tablets stress the need for forgiveness, and describe war as the immediate result of plague; surrounding clans are weakened by the plague and the entire social order is disrupted. This results in a pleading for forgiveness as well as a debate about the authority of the gods. There is dissent and disagreement about how to respond and, ultimately, who is in control:

> I am now continuing to make my plea to the Storm-god, my lord, concerning the plague. Hear me, O Storm-god, my lord, and save my life! [I say] to you [as follows]: The bird takes refuge in the cage, and the cage preserves its life. Or if something bothers some servant and he makes a plea to his lord, his lord listens to him, [has pity] on him, and he sets right what was bothering him. Or if some servant has committed a sin, but he confesses the sin before his lord, his lord may do with him whatever he wishes; but since he has confessed his sin before his lord, his lord's soul is appeased, and the lord will not call that servant to account. I have confessed the sin of my father. It is so. I have done it. If there is some restitution [to be made] – then there has already [been paid] much for this plague [caused by] the prisoners of war who were brought back from Egyptian territory and by the civilian captives who were brought back. [And] since Hatti has made restitution through the plague, it

[has made restitution] for it twenty-fold. Indeed, it has already become that much. And yet the soul of the Storm-god of Hatti, my lord, and of all the gods, my lords, is not at all appeased. Or if you want to require from me some additional restitution, specify it to me in a dream, and I shall give it to you.

(Singer 2002: 57–61)

Objects such as the 'Plague Prayers' tablets offer a wealth of meaning for humanities scholars, as they can enable us to draw parallels between the past and the present, examine modes of communication and explore the changing nature of human relationships, morals, conflicts and beliefs. Analyzing the content of these tablets, we can see that they not only provide us with an account of the plague, a description of civil unrest and subsequent war. We can also garner a sense of the politics of the period, the complex relationship between rulers and deities, and can explore the use of the tablet as a medium both for communication and public ritual. There is also a use of linguistic skill that can be discerned, where religious ritual becomes ingrained in a framework of the legal rhetoric of the time and the morals this enforces:

When I celebrated the festivals, I busied myself for all the gods. I did not pick out any single temple. I have repeatedly pled to all the gods concerning the plague, and I have repeatedly made vows [to them] saying: 'Listen [to me O gods], my [lords, and send away] the plague from Hatti. Hatti can [no longer bear this plague. Let the matter on account of which] it has been decimated [either be established through an oracle], or [let me see] it [in a dream, or let a man of god] declare [it].' But the gods [did not listen] to me, [and] the plague has not subsided in Hatti. [Hatti has been severely oppressed by the plague].

(Singer 2002: 57–61)

This structuring provides a sense of exchange, of giving and receiving in order to reduce the suffering of the time or to offset any culpability for causing the plague in the first place.

From this ancient example, we can immediately see beyond plagues as a medical concern and perceive their impact on people's way of life, on their belief systems, relationships and identities. Plagues form metaphors for how people live their lives and are deeply political in nature, both in the way in which societies seek to contain and curb the spread of infection and in the way in which people have responded to encounters with plague. This is as relevant today as it was 3000 years ago, as we continue to confront similar issues. The emergence of the COVID-19 pandemic in 2020 resulted in inevitable questions about who was to blame for both the emergence and the rapid spread of the virus, as the pandemic signalled a threat to human life, affecting people in different, yet devastating, ways. The spread of the virus acted as a form of plague which led to contrasting reactions and state interventions (or the lack of interventions), and to civil disobedience, as people felt a growing sense of diminishing freedom and a view that there was one rule for the elite and another for ordinary people. As well as their inevitable impact on world economies, these events triggered questions about different forms of power and control.

Plague as metaphor

Within this context, the humanities include fields of academic enquiry that, at face value, have played a backseat role in public debates about the impact of COVID-19, as the medical sciences took the front-and-centre stage in advising of effective ways of avoiding contact with the virus and in developing an effective vaccination to combat the disease. However, the humanities have a lot to say, not only about the effect of pandemics through time but also in offering insights into the broader social, cultural and political impacts of disease on society. The humanities have methods to gauge the ways in which plagues impact the workings of everyday lives and our relationships with each other, and they can also comment critically on the broader metaphors and meanings that emerge in a society riddled by plague. It is no surprise that historians, philosophers and cultural critics have been fascinated by human responses to crises through time but writers, artists, poets and musicians have also responded to plague in meaningful, creative ways. In her book *Illness as Metaphor*, for example, Susan Sontag stressed that any disease that is treated as a mystery and feared acutely enough by society will be felt to be morally, if not literally, contagious, and that metaphors attached to diseases imply 'living processes of a particularly resonant and horrid kind' (Sontag 1978: 2). Sontag describes the difference between epidemics that strike each person as part of an afflicted community and other diseases, such as tuberculosis, that were understood more as isolating people one by one from their community. As a pandemic, COVID-19 seemed to blend these conditions; afflicting entire communities, countries and continents yet seeming to affect individuals arbitrarily. Sontag argued that any disease that has a mysterious quality, or is 'multi-determined' in terms of origin and causes, carries with it a greater potential for metaphorical use, particularly in relation to what 'is felt to be socially or morally wrong' (Sontag 1978: 61). Metaphorical reactions to plague often stem from fear and a lack of understanding of the root causes of the disease. This results in psychological interpretations of disease where people develop ideas that their moral code, or a positive attitude, can overcome infection or rid individuals of disease. Sontag continues:

> In the plague-ridden England of the late sixteenth and seventeenth centuries [...] it was widely believed that 'the happy man would not get plague.' The fantasy that

a happy state of mind would fend off disease probably flourished for all infectious diseases, before the nature of infection was understood.

(Sontag 1978: 55)

Whilst these psychological understandings undermine the 'reality' of a disease, Sontag stresses that this form of psychologizing seems to offer people a form of control over experiences and events over which they, in fact, have little or no control. Whilst these forms of psychologizing perhaps can be related to the misinformed or to desperate citizens striving to find order amid chaos, it was surprising to see similar metaphors emerge from governments during the advent of the COVID-19 pandemic. For example, in the United Kingdom, the then British Prime Minister Boris Johnson adopted deeply problematic battle metaphors tied to the Second World War within his early speeches and COVID briefings (Musolff 2022). Moreover, when Johnson himself contracted the virus and was subsequently admitted to hospital, Johnson's political supporters argued that the Prime Minister would overcome the effects of the virus, mainly due to his heroic character (McCormick 2020). Here, the alignment with the Second World War battle metaphors and narratives of the hero overcoming adversity fed into much wider rhetorical processes linked to post-Brexit Britain and the cultivation of Johnson's own image as a classicist and as a politician who embodied the spirit of Winston Churchill. However, as a response to the pandemic alone, the sentiment that bravery and/or mental attitude could ward off the impact of the virus was incredibly ill-advised and offensive to so many people who had suffered at the hands of the disease.

The politics of plague

On a political level, the philosopher Michel Foucault suggested that the changing relationship to plague over time was directly related to changes in which systems of power and control are exercised (Foucault 2003). Foucault argued that changes in policy towards plagues in the seventeenth century resulted in a shift in the presentation of power. Rather than simply excluding plague victims from society, new forms of monitoring and surveillance were introduced in order to maintain order, and this ranged from the creation of plague towns to designated quarantine areas and regulations. In each case, Foucault suggested that these systems of monitoring and surveillance mirrored broader shifts in political systems and the need for a more coercive and consensual form of power and control. The emergence of COVID-19 brought a modern twist to plague metaphors as well as debates about political power and control. As with other plagues, COVID-19

INTRODUCTION

emerged as unfathomable at first, unaccountable in terms of its origins, and mysterious in the way in which it seemed to have a vastly different impact on different people. Indeed, while some people remained untouched following an encounter with COVID-19, others perished within days of contracting the virus. This unpredictable effect, as with other plagues, fed into broader metaphors about humanity and how we should live our lives. The subsequent roll-out of the vaccine programme also created additional layers of meaning and moral enquiry; from questions of political control and regulation to ethics and human rights. As a metaphor, the virus appeared to act as a sign of the times and, similar to the Hittite 'Plague Prayers' that opened this chapter, perhaps a deeper sense of humanity itself as being to blame for the emergence of the virus. For some, COVID-19 was interpreted as a by-product of the excesses of current human existence; of over-indulgent lifestyles and the destruction of the planet, bound up with debates about the Anthropocene; of the speed of human lifestyle; of cheap travel and recklessness in terms of sustainability and global carbon emissions; of a lack of care and understanding of environmental change, etc. (Wissenberg 2022). These excesses seemed to mirror the speed of contamination and the helplessness that ensued. COVID-19 could be regarded as a broader symptom of a culture that had assumed freedoms without responsibilities and the virus became a pathological space where disease spreads and proliferates, where people had to keep apart in order to remain safe; this, in turn, resulted in a change in attitude towards public spaces and places.

Encountering the plague

We argue that a broader engagement with historical change, meaning-making, comparative critical thinking and creativity through the lenses of different humanities subjects can inform debates and provide useful insights into human behaviour, and it is with this in mind that we conceived the idea for this collection. In conceiving *Encountering the Plague*, we started with the premise that the natural sciences can only go so far in accounting for the way in which people behave and relate to one another. Pandemics generate specific meanings and human behaviours that impact everyday lives and trigger emotional responses that go beyond scientific explanation. Scientific responses to pandemics also lead to a range of other social dilemmas that need to be discussed and evaluated; consider, for example, attitudinal differences to vaccination (which led to another series of societal problems and challenges, the questioning science, the clash between religious groups and the rationalistic position of science), regulations governing civil liberties, the suspicion regarding government contracts for personal protective equipment and the supply of pharmaceutical goods, the spread of fake news or suspicions about the role of 'Big Pharma' in a global marketplace.

This collection offers an opportunity to use the humanities as a lens to reflect on responses to plagues of the past and to explore specific challenges and conditions of the present day. In putting this collection together, we wanted to showcase the disparate voices that shape the humanities today; perspectives included in this collection draw on the fields of history, linguistics, media and cultural studies, theology, law, literary studies, archaeology and musicology. *Encountering the Plague* also serves as a showcase of work aligned with the Humanities in the European Research Area (HERA), a network whose joint Research Programmes have served as the primary support for the transnational research in the humanities in Europe since 2009.

As with the cuneiform tablets that were discussed at the opening of this chapter, the history of plague is often revealed through material objects. These material objects, whether in the form of written chronicles, artworks, stone carvings, poetry, songs or literature, are revelatory in what they tell us about mankind's response to crises, whether expressing anxiety about the present, using creativity to imagine a different future, or reflecting on the impact of the plague in the past. Since the mid-1980s and early 1990s, material culture has been of growing interest to a broader field of humanities scholars to the extent that the study of materiality pervades most disciplines, from history to anthropology, cultural and media studies to archaeology (Tilley et al. 2006; Hannan and Longhair 2017). Therefore, it is through reference to material objects (photographs, paintings, texts, etc.) that our contributors begin each chapter, exploring ways in which the history of plague can be opened up to allow for different disciplines to participate meaningfully in appraisals of the past and its relationship to the present. Each image connects to the theme of plague in some way or is used as a starting point for discussion. The images themselves offer meaningful ways to think about how identities are shaped through crises and how different communities have tackled plagues through time. We can think about lessons learned from the past and common themes that unite different plague moments in history; from the myth and belief in divine intervention – or punishment – to the realities of everyday life and the impact that plagues have on both individuals and communities. Some of the chosen objects serve as documents of plague, whilst others highlight creative responses. In each case, our contributors reflect on what these objects, and their broader social and political contexts, can tell us about civilization, the complexities of human life, and our shared resilience in times of crises.

We have divided this volume into four interconnected sections. The first examines the relationship between rituals and behaviour and the way in which the recent pandemic impacted attitudes and everyday life, from changes to religious rites to human rights challenges. Archaeologist Jo Sofaer opens this volume with an exploration of the role that heritage sites can play in countering anxiety caused by the pandemic. Drawing on a survey of visitors to Corfe Castle, Sofaer explores the need for escapism among groups and explores the relationship between people and place. Theologians Piotr Roszak and Piotr Paweł Orłowski examine the ways in which new ritual forms have emerged during the COVID-19 pandemic. This chapter discusses creative approaches to ritualization within the religious sphere, alongside the recalling of older traditions, such as the wearing of liturgical gloves, which emerged as a direct response to changing societal needs and state regulations. The chapter analyses the elements of the plague that have been ritualized in religious life alongside the recalling of practices and commitment signals, which provide opportunities to monitor others for sincerity. In the final chapter of this section, legal scholars Grażyna Baranowska and Aleksandra Gliszczyńska-Grabias pose the question of what makes people take part in large-scale protests during a pandemic and what motivates people to take risks in a time of plague. The chapter explores the tensions between rights to assembly and the actions of the state and explores both positive and negative aspects of human behaviour in pandemic times, as well as people's changing relationship to the law.

The second section of *Encountering the Plague* offers examples of encounters with the plague throughout history. Historian Charles Giry-Deloison presents a compelling study of experiences of the plague in London in the sixteenth and seventeenth centuries. The chapter compares two very different literary genres: a pamphlet (*The Wonderfull Yeare*) and a medical treatise (*Loimologia*), to examine two first-hand accounts of the plague. This is followed by medical historian and ethicist Florian Steger's examination of the way in which ancient texts encompass themes ranging from individual psychosocial reactions to disease, to political crises, economic downturns, and social instability. Steger questions what ancient texts can tell us today in terms of responses to the current pandemic. Finally, cultural historians James Brown and Gabrielle Robilliard examine how public space is understood as essential for public and community cohesion and well-being, and yet, reactions to the closure and control of public space have the potential to differ in fascinating ways according to time and place. Brown and Robilliard's chapter explores the relationship between plagues and public space and their analysis uses the past to inform current debates and tensions about the role of public space today.

Our third section explores the politics and discourse of COVID-19 through the analysis of different media texts. Arts and Media scholar Agnieszka Jelewska discusses the relationship between new technologies and knowledge production. She draws on the data visualizations that emerged during COVID-19 to discuss the gaps between expert knowledge, and broader social perceptions and understandings of the pandemic. In the following chapter, language and media expert Malgorzata Majewska offers an analysis of Polish media during the COVID-19 pandemic to explore the way meaning is constructed and conveyed within different media contexts, and how medical discourses were constructed and framed through language. This section concludes with linguistic and language scholars Rūta Petrauskaitė and Darius Amilevičius's exploration of the relationship between language and power through an analysis of the Lithuanian media during two years of the COVID-19 pandemic. Drawing on discourse analysis, their chapter evaluates the texts, language, style and stereotypes presented within mainstream media, and examines the wider social and political implications of these sources.

The final section of *Encountering the Plague* examines the relationship between creativity, cultural texts and plague, from the uses of art as a means of understanding the pandemic to creative responses to encountering lockdown. As an expert in Brazilian film, literature and culture, Sara Brandellero presents a reading of Kleber Mendonca Filho and Juliano Dornelles's 2019 film *Bacurau* as a way of examining questions of disease, unequal access to medical care, and state-sponsored necropolitics. Whilst the subject of study was filmed and released in pre-pandemic times, Brandellero explores the ways in which the creative output of the film resonates with the plight of millions under COVID-19. The following chapter by electronic literature specialists Anna Nacher, Søren Bro Pold and Scott Rettberg explores the aesthetics, narrativity and use of media in electronic literature and digital art related to COVID-19. The chapter documents creative responses within digital art and electronic literature (e-lit) through the presentation of interviews, exhibitions and presentations by artists from the Spring of 2020. In the final chapter of this section, Tony Whyton examines the way in which fictional accounts of plague can tell us much about the human experience of a pandemic. Examining the interrelationship between Albert Camus's 1947 novel *The Plague* and the blues song 'St James Infirmary', Whyton explores the way in which these texts meaningfully engage with human emotions and help people deal with encounters with plague. The chapter reiterates the importance of arts and culture in everyday life and examines creative ways of thinking about the arts and culture as they illuminate and reflect on the spread and proliferation of viruses. The volume concludes with a chapter by Wojciech Sowa who makes a powerful statement about the power of the humanities in times of crisis.

Encountering the Plague is not designed to provide an exhaustive take on the humanities and its relevance to plagues through time. Instead, we view this as a polemical collection designed to encourage readers to think about the relationship between past and present, from different humanities perspectives, and to consider COVID-19 as a starting point to think more broadly about plagues and the human condition. We encourage readers to engage with these contrasting texts as a way to think about everyday objects and experiences, and how they can open doors to the most profound issues and challenges during times of crisis.

NOTE

1. Cf., for example, the disastrous effects of the Black Death in Norway (1349–50), which led to a centuries long period of stagnation: losing its position as a major Kingdom in the Klamar Union and ultimately becoming a Danish province in 1536. Due to the plague, 60–65 per cent of the population died and the Norwegian elites suffered big losses. A report from 1351 to 1352 stated that the tax to the Pope was impossible to collect in Norway because the entire administration had broken down and a great lack of organization existed there because of the plague (Myrdal 2004).

REFERENCES

Foucault, Michel (2003), *Abnormal: Lectures at the College de France 1974–1975*, London and New York: Verso.

Hannan, Leonie and Longhair, Sarah (2017), *History Through Material Culture*, Manchester: Manchester University Press.

McCormick, Lisa (2020), 'Marking time in lockdown: Heroization and ritualization in the UK during the coronavirus pandemic', *American Journal of Cultural Sociology*, 8, pp. 324–51.

Musolff, Andreas (2022), '"World-beating" pandemic responses: Ironical, sarcastic, and satirical use of war and competition metaphors in the context of COVID-19 pandemic', *Metaphor and Symbol*, 37:2, pp. 76–87.

Myrdal, Janken (2004), 'Digerdöden, pestvågor och ödeläggelse Ett perspektiv på senmedeltidens Sverige', Uppsala, Avdelningen för agrarhistoria.

Singer, Itamar and Hoffner, Harry A. (2002), *Hittite Prayers*, Atlanta, GA: Society for Biblical Literature.

Sontag, Susan (1978), *Illness as Metaphor*, New York: Farrar, Straus & Giroux.

Tilley, Christopher, Keane, Webb, Kuchler, Susanne, Rowlands, Michael and Spyer, Patricia (eds) (2006), *Handbook of Material Culture*, London: Sage.

Wissenburg, Marcel (2022), 'The plague, the anthropocene, and Covid-19', in P. Mossleh (ed.), *Corona Phenomenon: Philosophical and Political Questions*, Leiden: Brill, pp. 215–21.

RITUALS AND RITES,
RIGHTS AND BEHAVIOURS

2

Heritage, Escapism and Anxiety: Visits to Corfe Castle during the COVID-19 Pandemic

Joanna Sofaer

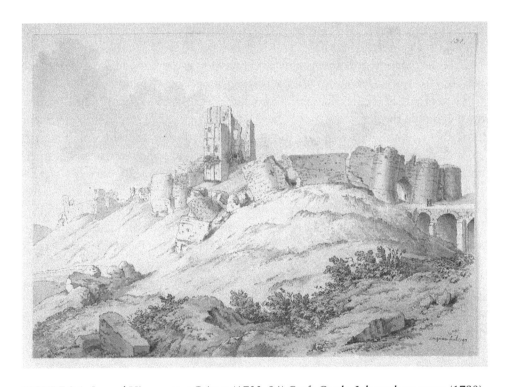

FIGURE 2.1: Samuel Hieronymus Grimm (1733–94) Corfe Castle. Ink wash on paper (1790). British Library f.131.

Heritage, anxiety and escapism

The COVID-19 pandemic was characterized by changes in the most fundamental aspects of human society. In the United Kingdom, the public health countermeasures that were imposed required significant cognitive and behavioural modifications in the way individuals lived their daily lives, altering interpersonal behaviours and social connections (O'Connor et al. 2021; Marroquin et al. 2020). So profound were these changes that Horesh and Brown (2020) have characterized COVID-19 as a mass trauma event. In the United Kingdom, estimates suggest that almost a quarter of the population experienced anxiety, with one-fifth experiencing clinically significant symptoms of anxiety and depression (Fancourt et al. 2020; O'Connor et al. 2021; Kwong et al. 2021; McPherson et al. 2021). These rates are considerably higher than those reported in UK samples before the pandemic (Arias-de la Torre et al. 2021; Löwe et al. 2008).

Escapism is a universal human mechanism that forms part of a strategy for coping with anxiety and stress (Evans 2014). It enables people to 'leave' the reality in which they live in a cognitive and emotional way (Vorderer 1996: 311). Common forms of positive escapism include reading, listening to music, exercising and gardening. However, escapism may also be detrimental, such as the use of drugs or excessive gaming (Melodia et al. 2020; Eden et al. 2020; Jouhki and Oksanen 2022). The outcomes of escapism depend on whether an individual is able to cope with the stressors adequately and the strategy employed (Melodia et al. 2020).

Lowenthal (2015: 105) suggests that when we cannot face today's news, 'rather than enhance the here and now, the past may replace the intolerable present altogether'. In this sense, an escape to the past may be part of a complex multifaceted emotional, cognitive and behavioural effort to 'manage specific external and/or internal demands that are seen as taxing or exceeding the resources of the person' (Lazarus and Folkman 1984: 141). Escape to the past can take many forms and, as with other forms of escapism, has the potential for both positive and negative effects. Pre-pandemic research on heritage and escapism has largely focused on escapism as a dimension of the experience economy and the attempt to escape the increasing homogenization of the world (Suntikul and Jachna 2016; Pine and Gilmore 1998; Radder et al. 2011; Kim and Jamal 2007; Laing and Crouch 2011; Gardiner et al. 2022), the use of new technologies such as augmented reality in museums and heritage settings (e.g. Han et al. 2021; Trunfio et al. 2022; Buoncontri and Marasco 2017) and nostalgia for an idealized version of the past, including visits to heritage places, the deployment of heritage as spectacle to distract from economic crisis and participation in re-enactment to escape a high-tech world and regain a sense of purpose (e.g. Lowenthal 2015; Fouseki and Dragouni 2017; Kelly 2009; MacCannell 1973). Although the experience economy and new technologies are understood in terms of visitor benefits, nostalgia is often seen as negative and, in some cases, even as dangerous. Thus, scholars have argued that nostalgic and sentimental views of the past as a 'golden age', which value the past more highly than the present, can provoke alienation and make it a hazardous place for the escapist to inhabit (Lowenthal 1985; Kelly 2009; Urry 1996; MacCannell 1992; Huyssen 2001; Hertzman et al. 2008).

In this chapter, I examine the role of escapism in visits to Corfe Castle, England, before and during the COVID-19 pandemic. Corfe Castle has been a visitor attraction for almost three centuries, establishing it as a place of escapism in the popular imagination. Although it is not possible to directly compare the responses of visitors during the COVID-19 pandemic with those of visitors before it, the long history of tourism at Corfe Castle offers some insights into potential continuity and change in perceptions and visitor experiences as a result of the encounter with COVID-19. Based on interview and survey data from 160 visitors to the site collected from June to October 2020 as part of the project *Places of Joy: Heritage After Lockdown*, I argue that visits to the site during the pandemic were part of a positive escapism coping strategy that was closely linked to visitors' wellbeing at a time of profound anxiety. I suggest that the expression of escapism varies over time and meets contextually specific needs that intersect with the deep history of the site in multiple ways and to different extents.

Corfe Castle as an escapist visitor attraction

Corfe Castle is an iconic ruin. Guarding a gap in the Purbeck Hills, it was built shortly after the Norman Conquest of England in 1066 and was partly demolished in 1646 during the English Civil War, following an Act of Parliament. From the eighteenth century to the present day, the site's rich history has increasingly been intertwined with its role as a visitor attraction and its place in the biographies of those who visit the site.

Corfe Castle first became a popular place to visit during the Georgian period. Travelling as a form of leisure was primarily experienced in the first half of the eighteenth century through the European Grand Tour. However, as travelling conditions in England improved from the 1770s and the Napoleonic Wars prevented travel to the continent, there was an increase in domestic tourism and interest in the countryside and local antiquities (Botto 2015; Dolman 2003). For example, the Swiss émigré Samuel Hieronymus Grimm (1733–94), travelled extensively throughout his adopted country in the late eighteenth century, capturing 'everything curious' for his patron Sir Richard Kaye, including Corfe Castle (Dolman 2003) (Figure 2.1). Travellers' guides drew attention to Corfe Castle as part of a 'British Grand Tour' (Wilson and Mackley 2000). *The Weymouth Guide* (1785) describes it as 'one of the finest ruins in Europe' (Delamotte 1785), while *Ryall's New Weymouth Guide* (1790) states, to thofe who have leifure and an inclination of viewing whatever is curious, I would recommend to them to vifit the ruins of Corfe Caftle, which makes fuch a figure in the Sazon Hisftory, – This once proud place in its priftine glory, muft have held its head above every other building in the neighbourhood, or perhaps in the Kingdom. –It is impoffible to view it even now, without thofe feelings which imrefs the mind with uncommon emotions. –The ponderous meffy fragments of disjointed walls, which feem ready to quit their apparent inadequate holds, ftrike you with terror! And the whole whether abftracted or collectively viewed, engages a ferious attention and fills the mind with aftonifhment! ... every ftep you go, you fee fomething to admire, fomething to ponder on.

(Love 1790: 52)

Such regional publications, as well as engravings and paintings, played an important role in the circulation of information about Corfe Castle. They provided proof that historical marvels and depth of civilization were to be found not only on the continent but also closer to home. Georgian guidebooks frequently emphasize wonder, astonishment and fear, encouraging the visitor to engage with these emotions. By the end of the period, these tropes appear to have been well established. Thus, *The Weymouth and Melcombe Regis New Guide* (1835) states:

The vast fragments of the king's tower, the round tower leaning as if ready to fall, the broken walls, and the huge mass hurled into the vale below, form such as scene of havoc and devastation, as must strike the spectator at once with horror and regret.

(Anon. 1835: 86)

By the Victorian period, the castle had become a popular day trip for visitors to the area. In 1882, Sir Edward Walter Hamilton visited the site and recorded in his diary:

Last Sunday, when at Swanage, we drove over to see Corfe Castle – the finest ruin I ever saw. The stonework is marvellous. It was destroyed in the Civil War, and the masonry is of such magnificent solidity that huge masses have fallen perfectly intact.

(Sir Edward Walter Hamilton 11 August 1882 [Bahlman n.d.])

In 1885, the construction of a branch line railway from Wareham made the nearby town of Swanage accessible by train, thereby facilitating Victorian visitors to the castle. Swanage become a seaside resort and Corfe Castle a 'must-see' attraction. The Victorian passion for travel saw a proliferation of guidebooks referring to the castle and photographs of the site in albums, books and magazines, such as Philip Brannon's (1860) *The Illustrated Historical and Picturesque Guide to Corfe*

Castle, Wareham, and the Antiquities of the Isle of Purbeck or *Swanage, Corfe Castle and Neighbourhood: The New Collotype Album of Picturesque Views* (Anon. 1890). Picnicking at the site was a popular activity in the Victorian period recorded in visitor's journals. For example, in 1875, Mary and Kate, sisters of the author Thomas Hardy, joined the Hardys (then in Swanage) for a picnic at the castle (Chalfont 1993). *A Descriptive Guide to Bournemouth, Christchurch, Wimborne and Corfe Castle* tells visitors that,

> Situated in the Isle of Purbeck, this ruin has always been an object of deep interest, and visitors to Bournemouth will find it affords an excellent day's 'outing', whether they seek a simple inspection of the magnificent ruins, or combine with it a pleasant picnic.
>
> (Hankinson 1891: 96)

Visits to the site formed part of a wider genre whereby Victorians created a psychological escape from everyday life by immersing themselves in exotic fictive worlds, often experienced vicariously through literature and paintings. Corfe featured in several of these, including Thomas Hardy's *The Hand of Ethelberta*, in which the heroine has a picnic at the 'notable ruin' of Corvesgate (Corfe Castle) (Lewer 1990; Elliott 1990).

In the spirit of Victorian moralism, people were encouraged to use the visit as an improving as well as enjoyable recreational experience. The same guide goes on to provide the visitor with an extended discussion of the history of the castle and a detailed description of the ruin itself, which combines didactic explanation, romantic aestheticism and moralism. Corfe's past was not a period desirable to hark back to, but rather one to learn lessons for the future. The entry to Corfe Castle ends by enjoining the reader to reflect on the sacrifice of the building and suffering within it:

> before us rise majestically the lofty fragments of the Great Keep, or Kings Tower; the south front, and the adjoining returns of the two side walls, and the east side or pillar like portion isolated from the return, alone remains standing, enveloped in thick ivy. Beautiful is the contrast of this noble column of rich verdure with the light varied grey and moss-grown walls of the other sides of the keep [...] We cannot but regret that the exigencies of the times appear to have rendered so complete a destruction of the fine old edifice necessary: the blow struck at the feudal system paved the way to our present freedom. Possibly we may be more reconciled to the sacrifice when we think of the sufferings, long and bitter, which hundreds of prisoners endured within these walls, long lingering misery ended only by death.
>
> (Hankinson 1891: 106–07)

Similarly, a guidebook from 1857 gives a short history of the castle and then concludes:

> We recount these deeds to show the spirit and conduct of times happily passed away. These beautiful ruins bear not the guilt of those perpetrations; and in them, it may be, is set forth a moral lesson, safe to learn and good to practise: hence, in contemplating the ruins of Corfe Castle, we may realize that there are 'sermons in stones'.
> (Archer 1857: n.pag.)

By the early twentieth century, accounts of visits to the castle had shifted in tone. Allan Brown, an Australian soldier training at Wareham in 1916, wrote in his diary that Corfe is 'a very ancient castle which we read about in the history books at school [...] I visited this place a few times, as I fell in love with the old fashioned little village' (Brown 1916–17: 78–79 in White 2014). White (2014: 6) identifies the visit as nostalgia linked to a soldier's homesickness: Corfe represents a personal memory that allows tourists to link their experience of Britain's past with their own memories of younger days.

After the First World War, Corfe Castle became a stop on motor tours along the south coast (e.g. Brilliant 1925). Following the Second World War, an increase in car ownership and disposable income contributed to the development of mass tourism in the area. This coincided with national moves following the Second World War to preserve buildings of special architectural or historical interest established in the Town and Country Planning Acts of 1944 and 1947. The desire to both create and preserve a national heritage collection took expression through a survey by the Ministry of Housing and Local Government, which created the National Heritage List for England (Hunter 1996; Thurley 2013). This pioneering survey took nearly 25 years and produced 120,000 entries on the list, including Corfe Castle, which was listed on 20 November 1959. The government also started to intervene in tourism, recognizing the economic importance of the tourist industry in the 1969 Development of Tourism Act, which set up the British Tourist Authority (now Visit Britain) and the English Tourist Board (now VisitEngland) (Middleton and Lickorish 2007). In 1982, the castle passed from private ownership under the Bankes family and was given to the National Trust as a gift to the nation. These legislative developments and changes in ownership shifted the status of Corfe Castle towards public recognition as a 'heritage site'. Corfe became an essential family day trip from the seaside – a hedonistic escape and a place of release from daily life immortalized on postcards and in family albums.

The castle's status as a 'heritage site' was augmented by more than a decade of archaeological excavation which took place from the mid-1980s. Data from these excavations were integrated into the presentation of the site with interpretation boards provided at key locations to assist visitor learning. Preservation of the castle also became a priority in order to retain the ruin, despite questions over the £700,000 price tag (Reynolds 2006).

> It does sound a lot of money to keep it as a ruin, but it's such an important ruin. It's so romantic and an absolute icon of British castles [...] All thoughts of rebuilding were banished as heresy long ago. In 1715, one of the Bankes family did some drawings of how he'd like to restore it in a slightly Gothic way. Fortunately, nothing happened because it is an absolutely magical place as it is and you can see more how it was built now than if it was restored.
> (Pam White, Corfe Castle Community Learning Officer in Reynolds 2006)

The 2019 National Trust Handbook describes Corfe Castle as a 'fairytale fortress' that is:

> a favourite haunt for adults and children alike – all ages are captivated by these romantic ruins with their breathtaking views. There are 1,000 years of the castle's history as a royal palace and fortress to be discovered here. Fallen walls and secret places tell tales of treachery and treason around every corner.
> (National Trust 2019: 52)

It promises 'an action-packed programme of fun family history events', accompanied by an image of re-enactors of the Civil War, a romantic photograph of a woman standing alone under an arch and a dramatic aerial shot of the site set in the surrounding landscape (National Trust 2019: 52–53). Thus, education was joined to romanticism. In 2015, National Trust volunteers built a replica trebuchet that remains in the castle today as a way of helping 'to bring the medieval past to life' (Durkin 2015). 'Edutainment' in the form of dressing up, the obligatory photo of the visitor in Medieval stocks and re-enactment events took prominent roles in site promotion. Not only was Corfe Castle a place to take family, friends and children on a fun day out, but narrative and storytelling became part of the visitor experience, stimulating imagination about the past. As with many other heritage sites, Corfe became a nostalgic space where it was easy for visitors to vicariously experience the past, idealize it and indulge themselves in looking for the lost meanings of the present in a 'golden age' (Kelly 2009; Lowenthal 2015).

In the year prior to the COVID-19 pandemic (2019/20), Corfe Castle was one of the National Trust's most visited sites; it had more than a quarter of a million visitors (National Trust 2020). However, like other heritage destination sites in England, on 23 March 2020, Corfe Castle closed its doors as a result of the first national COVID-19 lockdown. Strict limits were imposed on daily life as people were ordered to only leave the house for essentials such as food, medicine exercise or to care for a vulnerable person. All non-essential shops were closed and gatherings of more than two people were banned. Tourism suddenly stopped and people were unable to visit. Peregrine falcons nested in the castle.

Escapism, psychological distance and visits to Corfe Castle during the COVID-19 pandemic

Corfe Castle reopened in June 2020. As an open-air site, it was part of the first phase of National Trust sites to open (Wilson 2020), but without its usual programme of interpretive activities. Instead, the site carefully regulated visitor numbers, required strict social distancing and imposed set visitor routes, the latter tastefully marked out with bunting so as to give the impression of a fete rather than a public health measure (Figure 2.2). This was a period of heightened anxiety caused by fear of infection, social isolation, loneliness, grief and financial worries. In this atmosphere, the opening up of society and visits to heritage sites, including Corfe Castle, took on particular significance. They were framed by self-awareness of why such visits took place (Sofaer et al. 2021), including the importance of escapism, which was facilitated by the unique time depth offered by the site.

The Places of Joy survey found that visitors to Corfe Castle reported levels of anxiety similar to those in the population at large during the summer and autumn of 2020 (Gallou et al. 2022). Seventy-nine per cent of participants said that visiting the site gave them an extremely or very strong sense of freedom and 27 per cent of participants explicitly identified a motive for visiting as 'To escape from the worry and boredom of COVID-19'. The importance of escapism also emerges in the thematic analysis of interview and free-text survey responses of visitors to the site, which are striking in their repeated use of the word 'escape' and related words such as 'release' and 'freedom' as a means of describing visitor experiences. Visitors to Corfe Castle experienced and reported escapism through their visit in four distinct but inter-related ways that could be felt both separately and together.

Geographical escape

The COVID-19 lockdown confined people to their homes and imposed national and international travel restrictions. It shrank people's worlds, recalibrating scales of geographical distance, and returned them to a time before aviation and mass transport. Travel is itself a form of positive escapism and may be a means to reprioritize and reorganize identities (Smith 2003). Seaton (2002: 162) describes tourism as being 'as much a quest to *be* as a quest to see', while Craik (1997: 114)

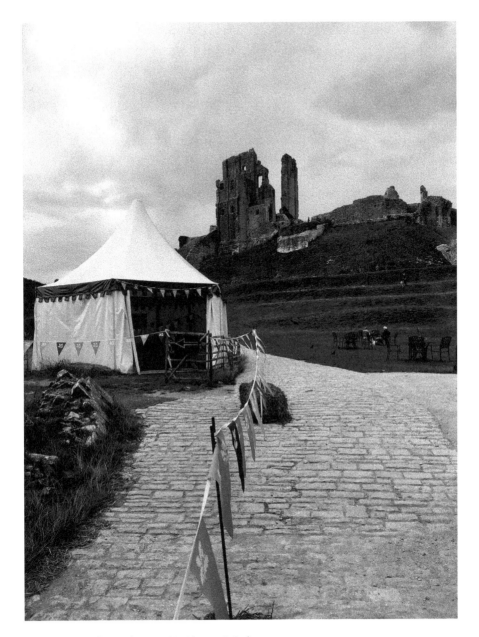

FIGURE 2.2: Corfe Castle in 2020. Photo: J. Sofaer.

suggests that 'Tourists revel in the otherness of destinations, people and activities because they offer the illusion or fantasy of otherness, of difference and counterpoint to the everyday.'

Travel requires a destination and, when the opportunity for limited travel returned, journeys to places in the United Kingdom, including Corfe Castle, became a place of escape; 49 per cent of the sample agreed that the visit was 'a change of scene'. As open-air heritage sites were amongst the first places to open (in a reduced field of options) and also perceived to be safer than indoor venues, Corfe Castle and other open-air sites became desirable destinations. In this sense, while some have argued that the escapist nature of physical travel has, to some extent, been replaced by virtual experiences or 'de-differentiated' from everyday experience (Smith 2003; Feifer 1985; Urry 1990; Walsh 1992), enforced travel restrictions during the pandemic may have reignited the explicit desire for travel as a form of escape from lockdown routines and as a means of reconstituting the self through engagement with the past as a form of otherness. Travel gained a new poignancy and thus visits to heritage sites took on meaning in and of itself (see also Sofaer et al. 2021).

This link between travel and visits to Corfe Castle was clearly articulated by a couple who were caravanning in the area:

> We have visited Corfe today on holiday from Cheshire. We have been before and absolutely love it. We missed be able to visit places to visit during lockdown. We're so glad to be able to go out again and escape the house. We have a caravan and like to visit different National Trust places around the country. We have the freedom to decide where to go.
>
> (Interview Corfe Castle July 2020)

Other interviewees indicated that visits to the site were part of a new type of 'staycation' rather than going abroad. Visits to heritage sites in England took the place of foreign travel. 'We have cancelled six holidays. We should be in the Canaries right now. We are [...] doing more in England and visiting historic places as part of our holiday in ways that we didn't before' (Interview Corfe Castle September 2020).

However, for some visitors, the visit held meaning precisely because of Corfe Castle's familiarity. Instead of going somewhere new, the release of lockdown allowed them to regain access to a meaningful place: 'This place has longstanding memories for me. Lovely to be able to visit again. Feel close to family members no longer here' (Survey Corfe Castle August 2020).

Temporal escape

The unique time depth of the heritage environment facilitated the illusion of a pre-pandemic space (Sofaer et al. 2021). Visits to Corfe Castle enabled people to move outside a COVID present into a pre-COVID past by visiting a place associated with a pre-pandemic environment. This temporal escape was often described in terms of a reminder of when life was 'normal' – the immediate period before the pandemic – rather than a deeper historical past. In this form of escape, time was related to geography and 'people step out of the present into the past of their choice' (Spender 1974 in Lowenthal 2015: 106). 'Coming here has really helped me gain a sense of normality' (Survey Corfe Castle 06.09.2020).

In the context of COVID-19, although heritage sites were objectively no safer than other open-air spaces, they were often perceived to be less dangerous. This may relate to a wider notion of the past as a safe place, as noted by Lowenthal (2015), who suggests that the past is 'safer' than the future and the present because it is perceived as fixed, known and thus reliable. The time depth of Corfe Castle facilitated a link between time and space such that safety became an important feature of escapism. 'I was bedridden for 3 months with COVID-19 in isolation. It is great to be able to get out and enjoy safe spaces like this' (Survey Corfe Castle 02.08.2020).

However, in contrast to analyses immediately before the pandemic, which tend to implicate specific histories of heritage sites in feelings of nostalgia for an ideal past and identify these as important to escapism at heritage destinations (Lowenthal 2015), relatively few visitors to Corfe Castle identified this as part of their experience. Although 50 per cent of survey respondents reported that their visit made them feel extremely or very nostalgic, this was overwhelmingly articulated in terms of nostalgia for pre-pandemic visits to the site with friends and family, and the perceived need to maintain a tradition of visits, rather than nostalgia for a deeper past or golden age. Furthermore, when asked why they had visited a heritage site instead of another form of public space, such as the park or the beach, although interviewees expressed curiosity about the place and an interest in history, longing for the deep past was conspicuously absent. Instead, visitors reflected on the deep past as a period of struggle. Nostalgia was replaced by a sense of identification with people in the past who had also overcome adversity. The survival of people in the past offered hope and ontological security in the present (Sofaer et al. 2021). Visitors had a strong awareness that medicine in the past was not as effective as in the present. 'The castle lasted. You'll last too!' (Interview Corfe Castle 02.08.2020). 'You wouldn't want to get sick in the Medieval times. COVID is frightening enough now' (Interview Corfe Castle 02.08.2020).

Social escape

In June 2020, just over a quarter of the UK population (26 per cent) reported feeling lonely (Office of National Statistics 2020). After a prolonged period of isolation, people were keen to escape the confines of their own company and to see friends and family. Heritage sites became important social spaces. Data from the Heritage After Lockdown project found that 79 per cent of visitors went to Corfe Castle to spend time with friends and family, compared to 42.4 per cent of visitors citing this as a reason to visit heritage sites before the pandemic (DCMS 2019. Taking Part Survey Year 14: England Adult Report (2018/19), cited in Historic England 2020: 33). Sharing the experience of the visit with other people was an important quality of this social experience; 50 per cent of respondents explicitly stated that they chose to visit in order to share their experience with others and 66 per cent of visitors said that their visit made them feel extremely or very connected with other people. 'I haven't seen the grandchildren for 6 months. They live in Aberdeen and London. We really missed them. We're all here for the weekend. It's great to get out of the house and a lovely place to meet up' (Interview Corfe Castle 18.06.20).

Bringing a picnic to the site and eating together were often important to the social nature of the visit. Many pubs and restaurants were closed and people were concerned about meeting indoors. Thus, picnics became a popular alternative, reviving a Victorian tradition at the site.

Experiential escape

Myth and fantasy play an important role in the social construction of visits to tourist sites (Rojek 1997). Visitors to Corfe Castle used the experience as a means of imagining hypothetical alternatives to the present reality. This took two distinct forms. The first involved imagining past worlds rather than wanting to actively return to them. This included, for example, putting oneself in the place of an inhabitant of the castle and wondering what it would be like to live there in winter or reflecting on how grand the structure must have been before it was destroyed. However, such reflections tended to verge on the mundane rather than reflecting the wonder of the Georgian period or Victorian romanticism. 'This is an amazing place but it must have been cold to live there. I can imagine it was freezing in winter' (Interview Corfe Castle 18.07.2020).

The second involved imagining a post-covid future. Here, the visit facilitated consideration of possibilities for life after lockdown, including thinking about personal lifestyle changes or imagining what changes the pandemic would make to a future world.

> For me, the lockdown helped to re-centre what is important in my life. Yes, it's been so challenging and frightening, and continues to be so, but I have personally discovered more about life closer to home and changed for the better many aspects of my life which has enhanced wellbeing.
>
> (Survey Corfe Castle 18.07.2020)

I don't feel that I need to travel abroad now. Discovering new places to visit in England has been a real benefit. And it's better for the planet. Maybe this experience will change things for the better.

(Interview Corfe Castle 06.09.2020)

Such future-focused thinking was more frequent than that linked to the imagination of the past. This raises the possibility that the experience of the pandemic may have re-orientated visitor responses. Unlike Victorian reactions to the site, this future focus was not moralistic in terms of learning from the past for the future. Instead, reflections on the visit were linked to expressions of hope for a post-pandemic world and better times to come.

Psychological distance and escapism

The concept of psychological distance provides a framework for understanding the effects of heritage tourism (Scarpi and Raggiotto 2023) and thus the origin and effects of escapism. Perceptions of psychological distance are closely tied to people's emotions, risk assessment and behavioural attitudes (Blauza et al. 2021; Wong et al. 2022). Recent research suggests that psychological distancing may offer avenues for adaptation and healthier coping at times of stress (Bowen 2021). It is therefore critical to wellbeing, where wellbeing is understood as 'how people feel and how they function, both on a personal and a social level, and how they evaluate their lives as a whole' (Michaelson et al. 2012: 6).

Psychologically distant things are those that are not present in the direct experience of reality, whereas those that are psychologically close are part of the reality of lived experience (Liberman et al. 2007; Liberman and Trope 2008). The concept of psychological distance thus provides a means of understanding the extent to which people's perception of objects and events is concrete (close) or abstract (distant) (McDonald et al. 2015) and forms the basis of construal level theory (CLT) (Trope and Liberman 2010). CLT suggests that while the construal of concrete constructs is focused on the details, that of more abstract constructs is concentrated on the big picture (McDonald et al. 2015), though these are on a scale rather than absolute opposites. Recent research suggests that psychological distancing may offer avenues for adaptation and healthier coping at times of stress (Bowen 2021).

Psychological distance is composed of four dimensions: Spatial distance refers to spatially remote locations (e.g. the South Pole or a place I go on holiday). Temporal distance refers to objects or events that may belong to the past or the future (e.g. the English Civil War or my year of retirement). Social distance refers to the experiences of other people (e.g. the way another person perceives the present situation). Hypothetical (experiential) distance refers to alternatives to reality – what could or might have been but never actually happened (e.g. what might have occurred had I married another person or if I had lived in Roman Britain) (Liberman et al. 2007). These dimensions are sensitive to cultural context and personal experience and provide a means of understanding people's perceptions of events (Maiella et al. 2020).

The dimensions of psychological distance can be used to understand escapism as a universal human phenomenon over time and space, with particular utility for understanding escapist responses to the COVID-19 pandemic. They map closely to the four forms of escapism experienced by visitors to Corfe Castle during the COVID-19 pandemic. The geographical escapism reported by visitors to Corfe Castle can be understood in terms of the construction of spatial distance. In relation to tourism, Ponsignon et al. (2021) suggest that the greater the perception of spatial distance, the greater the escapism, hedonic value and satisfaction with the tourism experience. Temporal escapism can be considered a means of removing oneself from the stress of the present by using the time depth of the site to create the illusion of temporal distance from the present reality of the pandemic. Experiential escape can be understood in terms of imaginative engagement with the history of place, which facilitates hypothetical (experiential) distancing from the reality of the COVID present. CLT indicates that in this process of *increasing* psychological distance, the pandemic became more abstract and people less focused on stressful day-to-day details. This suggests a mechanism by which visitors' use of the time depth and ruinous aesthetic of Corfe Castle acted as a positive behavioural adaptation at a time of stress and anxiety.

By contrast, in seeking release from the isolation of lockdown, the social escape and shared experience described by visitors to Corfe Castle can be understood as a deliberate attempt to *reduce* social distance. Despite its role in supporting public health during the pandemic, a growing body of evidence suggests the negative psychological consequences of social distancing (e.g. Ford 2020; Killgore et al. 2020; Marroquin et al. 2020; Tull et al. 2020). Visits to Corfe Castle can be identified as a positive behavioural response which involves a process of drawing closer to others and a concrete construal of shared experiences (see Bowen 2021). This was facilitated by the decision to engage socially with others through being in the same space as people with a shared interest or by using the castle as a meeting place for family and friends (see Sofaer et al. 2021). In some cases, this was accompanied by a reduction in geographical distance as people regained access to a place they had missed during lockdown. Here, the concrete construal of the site though a physical visit created a sense of comfort and familiarity.

Psychological distancing forms part of an adaptive emotion regulation toolkit that has been uniquely associated with a reduction in stress during the COVID-19 pandemic (Dicker et al. 2022). This also appears to be the case for visitors to Corfe Castle. Visitors reported statistically significant increases in positive affect and a reduction in negative affect following a visit (Gallou et al. 2022), suggesting that escapism as a means of psychological distancing was a positive mechanism for coping with stress during the pandemic.

Escapism before and during the COVID-19 pandemic

Escape to the past is not new and is deeply embedded within western culture (Lowenthal 2015). The long history of tourism at Corfe Castle is part of this history of escapism. It offers insights into potential continuity and change in use, perception and visitor experiences at the site, including as a result of the encounter with COVID-19. From the Georgian period to the present, the unique time depth and ruinous aesthetic of the site have facilitated escapism, but the cultural tropes associated with the site and the context of visits vary. Visits in the Georgian period were linked to a sense of wonder; the Victorians constructed their visits around romanticism, leisure and moral learning; experiences in the first half of the twentieth century were characterized by personal nostalgia followed by hedonism in the aftermath of war; and the period immediately prior to the COVID-19 pandemic can be understood in terms of education and vicarious nostalgia. By contrast, visits during the pandemic were articulated in terms of an explicit awareness of a suite of personal needs following a period of lockdown, including geographical, temporal, social and experiential escape. Although these may also have informed responses to the site before the pandemic, and it is difficult to directly compare historical pre-pandemic visitor experiences from guidebooks and diaries with visitor interviews and survey data collected during the pandemic, the largely present and future-focused responses of visitors suggest that experience of lockdown may have re-framed experiences of the site. In particular, visitor responses reveal the role of visits to the site in facilitating fundamental human needs as part of coping strategies during the pandemic. It is therefore possible to suggest shifts in the qualities of escapism experienced by visitors to Corfe Castle as a result of the encounter with COVID-19.

Lowenthal (2015) suggests that the designation of places as 'heritage sites' distinguishes and sets them apart from other places as 'islands of the past' that 'serve as refuges from modernity' (Lowenthal 2015: 108). This pre-pandemic analysis articulates 'refuge' in terms of nostalgia or a longing for the past that requires 'unawareness' and idealizes the past (Lowenthal 2015). In other words, it requires a particular understanding of the site as different from the present rather than as part of it. Although such 'unawareness' may be a necessary part of escapism – no one wants to escape to a time or place that is worse than their own – the implication that escapism is bound up with the *history of the site* being in some way preferable to the present does not align with the experiences of visitors to Corfe Castle during the COVID-19 pandemic. Instead, consumption of the past through visits to Corfe Castle was not generally related to an idealized or grand history of the site but was more frequently linked to the personal biographies of visitors. This did not require stepping back into the deep past of the castle but was often linked to memories of a much more recent personal past – a time of 'normality' before 23 March 2020. In doing so, escapism allowed people to cope with the uncertainty of the present. It also created an opportunity for visitors to reflect on their hopes for a better future.

Escapism at Corfe Castle was a positive means of coping with the unique stressors of the pandemic. This was not a matter of running away from modernity but rather a way of finding sanctuary within it. The site created the conditions for visitors to psychologically distance themselves from the pandemic in ways that responded to personal needs following an extended period of lockdown by drawing together a complex suite of temporal strands linking past, present and future. As a place of escape, Corfe Castle was woven into the twenty-first-century encounter with the plague.

REFERENCES

Anon. (1835), *The Weymouth and Melcombe Regis New Guide*, Weymouth: E. Groves.

Anon. (1890), *Swanage, Corfe Castle and Neighbourhood: The New Collotype Album of Picturesque Views*, n.p.

Archer, D. (1857), *Weymouth as a Watering Place. With a Description of the Town and Neighbourhood, the Breakwater and Its Construction, the Portland Quarries, the Chesil Beach, etc. etc., for the Use of Intending and Actual Visitor*, London: Simpkin and Marshall.

Arias-de la Torre, J., Vilagut, G., Ronaldson, A., Serrano-Blanco, A., Martín, V., Peters, M., Valderas, J. M., Dregan, A. and Alonso, J. (2021), 'Prevalence and variability of current depressive disorder in 27 European countries: A population-based study', *The Lancet Public Health*, 6:10, pp. e729–38.

Bahlman, D. W. R. (ed.) (n.d.), *The Diary of Sir Edward Walter Hamilton 1880–1885*, 1, New York: Oxford University Press, 2022 [online], pp. 1880–82, https://www.oxfordscholarlyeditions.com/display/10.1093/actrade/9780198815709.book.1/actrade-9780198815709-div2-352?rskey=Vnd2Zj&result=1. Accessed 25 March 2023.

Blauza, S., Heuckmann, B., Kremer, K. and Büssing, A. G. (2021), 'Psychological distance towards COVID-19: Geographical and hypothetical distance predict attitudes and mediate knowledge', *Current Psychology*, 42:10, pp. 1–12.

Botto, M. I. D. (2015), 'Garden tourism in England: An early discovery', in A. D. Rodrigues (ed.), *Gardens and Tourism for and Beyond Economic Profit*, Evora: CHAIA/CIUHCT, pp. 11–26.

Bowen, J. D. (2021), 'Psychological distance and the pandemic: Insights from construal level theory and relationship science', *Social and Personality Psychology Compass*, 5, p. e12594, https://doi.org/10.1111/spc3.12594.

Brannon, P. (1860), *The Illustrated Historical and Picturesque Guide to Corfe Castle, Wareham, and the Antiquities of the Isle of Purbeck*, London: R. Sydenham, Longman & Co.

Brilliant, M. (1925), Papers and Photographs of Mortimer Brilliant (1895–c.1990), University of Southampton Special Collections.

Brown, A. D. (1916–17), *Diary, 7 January 1916–3 November 1917*. ML MSS 17.

Buonincontri, P. and Marasco, A. (2017), 'Enhancing cultural heritage experiences with smart technologies: An integrated experiential framework', *European Journal of Tourism Research*, 17, pp. 83–101.

Chalfont, F. (1993), 'Hardy's residences and lodgings: Part two', *The Thomas Hardy Journal*, 9:1, pp. 41–61.

Craik, J. (1997), 'The culture of tourism', in C. Rojek and J. Urry (eds), *Touring Cultures. Transformations of Travel and Theory*, London: Routledge, pp. 123–46.

Delamotte, P. (1785), *The Weymouth Guide*, Weymouth: Frontiers Media.

Dicker, E. E., Jones, J. S. and Denny, B. T. (2022), 'Psychological distancing usage uniquely predicts reduced perceived stress during the COVID-19 pandemic', *Frontiers in Psychology*, 13, 838507, https://doi.org/10.3389/fpsyg.2022.838507

Dolman, B. (2003), '"Everything Curious": Samuel Hieronymus Grimm and Sir Richard Kaye', *Electronic British Library Journal*, https://bl.iro.bl.uk/concern/articles/3c65f3e3-fe63-416d-8b4b-fb79c515f4b0?locale=en. Accessed 25 March 2023.

Durkin, J. (2015), 'Trebuchet replica built at Corfe Castle', *Bournemouth Echo*, 27 June, https://www.bournemouthecho.co.uk/news/13356779.watch-trebuchet-replica-built-at-corfe-castle/. Accessed 25 March 2023.

Eden, A. L., Johnson, B. K., Reinecke, L. and Grady, S. M. (2020), 'Media for coping during COVID-19 social distancing: Stress, anxiety, and psychological well-being', *Frontiers in Psychology*, 11, p. 3388.

Elliott, R. (1990), 'Hardy and the middle ages', *The Thomas Hardy Journal*, 6:2, pp. 97–108.

Evans, A. (2014), *This Virtual Life. Escapism and Simulation in our Media World*, London: Fusion Press.

Fancourt, D., Steptoe, A. and Bu, F. (2020), 'Trajectories of anxiety and depressive symptoms during enforced isolation due to COVID-19 in England: A longitudinal observational study', *The Lancet Psychiatry*, 8:2, pp. 141–49.

Feifer, M. (1985), *Going Places. The Ways of the Tourist from Imperial Rome to the Present Day*, London: MacMillan.

Ford, M. B. (2020), 'Social distancing during the COVID-19 pandemic as a predictor of daily psychological, social, and health-related outcomes', *The Journal of General Psychology*, 148:3, pp. 249–71.

Fouseki, K. and Dragouni, M. (2017), 'Heritage spectacles: The case of Amphipolis excavations during the Greek economic crisis', *International Journal of Heritage Studies*, 23:8, pp. 742–58.

Gallou, E., Uzzell, D. and Sofaer, J. (2022), 'Perceived place qualities, restorative effects and self-reported wellbeing benefits of visits to heritage sites: Empirical evidence from a visitor survey in England', *Wellbeing, Space and Society*, 3, p. 100106.

Gardiner, S., Vada, S., Chiao Ling Yang, E., Khoo, C. and Le, T. H. (2022), 'Recreating history: The evolving negotiation of staged authenticity in tourism experiences', *Tourism Management*, 91, p. 104515.

Han, S., Yoon, J. H. and Kwon, J. (2021), 'Impact of experiential value of augmented reality: The context of heritage tourism', *Sustainability*, 13:8, p. 4147.

Hankinson, C. J. [Holland, C. Pseud] (1891), *A Descriptive Guide to Bournemouth, Christchurch, Wimborne and Corfe Castle*, 10th ed., Bournemouth: British Library Historical Print Editions.

Hertzman, E., Anderson, D. and Rowley, S. (2008), 'Edutainment heritage tourist attractions: A portrait of visitors' experiences at Storyeum', *Museum Management and Curatorship*, 23:2, pp. 55–175.

Historic England (2020), *Heritage and Society*, https://historicengland.org.uk/content/heritage-counts/pub/2020/heritage-and-society-2020/. Accessed 25 March 2023.

Horesh, D. and Brown, A. D. (2020), 'Traumatic stress in the age of COVID-19: A call to close critical gaps and adapt to new realities', *Psychological Trauma: Theory, Research, Practice, and Policy*, 12:4, pp. 331–35.

Hunter, M. (1996), *Preserving the Past: The Rise of Heritage in Modern Britain*, Stroud: Sutton.

Huyssen, A. (2001), 'Present pasts: Media, politics, amnesia', *Public Culture*, 12:1, pp. 21–38.

Jouhki, H. and Oksanen, A. (2022), 'To get high or to get out? Examining the link between addictive behaviors and escapism', *Substance Use & Misuse*, 57:2, pp. 202–11.

Kelly, C. (2009), 'Heritage', in R. Kitchin and N. Thrift (eds), *International Encyclopaedia of Human Geography*, London: Elsevier, pp. 91–97.

Killgore, W. D. S., Cloonan, S. A., Taylor, E. C., Lucas, D. A. and Dailey, N. S. (2020), 'Loneliness during the first half-year of COVID-19 lockdowns', *Psychiatry Research*, 294, pp. 113551–52.

Kim, H. and Jamal, T. (2007), 'Touristic quest for existential authenticity', *Annals of Tourism Research*, 34:1, pp. 181–201.

Kwong, A. S., Pearson, R. M., Adams, M. J., Northstone, K., Tilling, K., Smith, D., Fawns-Ritchie, C., Bould, H., Warne, N., Zammit, S. and Gunnell, D. J. (2021), 'Mental health before and during the COVID-19 pandemic in two longitudinal UK population cohorts', *The British Journal of Psychiatry*, 218:6, pp. 334–43.

Laing, J. and Crouch, G. (2011), 'Frontier tourism: Retracing mythic journeys', *Annals of Tourism Research*, 38:4, pp. 1516–34.

Lazarus, R. S. and Folkman, S. (1984), *Stress, Appraisal, and Coping*, New York: Springer.

Lewer, D. (1990), *Hardy in Swanage: 1875 and 'The Hand of Ethelberta' by Thomas Hardy*, Somerset: Dorset Publishing Company.

Liberman, N. and Trope, Y. (2008), 'The psychology of transcending the here and now', *Science*, 322:5905, pp. 1201–05.

Liberman, N., Trope, Y. and Stephan, E. (2007), 'Psychological distance', in A. W. Kruglanski and E. T. Higgins (eds), *Social Psychology: Handbook of Basic Principles*, New York: The Guilford Press, pp. 353–81.

Love, J. (1790), *New Weymouth Guide. A New Improved Weymouth Guide: Containing a Description of Weymouth, Portland, Lulworth Castle, and Every Place in the Neighbourhood Worth the Observation of Strangers. With a list of Lodging Houses. Embellished with a View of the Bay*, https://wellcomecollection.org/works/r6efytnx. Accessed 03 June 2024.

Löwe, B., Decker, O., Müller, S., Brähler, E., Schellberg, D., Herzog, W. and Herzberg, P. Y. (2008), 'Validation and standardization of the Generalized Anxiety Disorder Screener (GAD-7) in the general population', *Medical Care*, 46:3, pp. 266–74.

Lowenthal, D. (1985), *The Past Is a Foreign Country*, New York: Cambridge University Press.

Lowenthal, D. (2015), *The Past Is a Foreign Country-Revisited*, Cambridge: Cambridge University Press.

MacCannell, D. (1973), 'Staged authenticity: Arrangements of social space in tourist settings', *American Journal of Sociology*, 79:3, pp. 589–603.

MacCannell, D. (1992), *Empty Meeting Grounds: The Tourist Papers*, London: Routledge.

Maiella, R., La Malva, P., Marchetti, D., Pomarico, E., Di Crosta, A., Palumbo, R., Cetara, L., Di Domenico, A. and Verrocchio, M. C. (2020), 'The psychological distance and climate change: A systematic review on the mitigation and adaptation behaviors', *Frontiers in Psychology*, 11, p. 568899.

Marroquín, B., Vine, V. and Morgan, R. (2020), 'Mental health during the COVID-19 pandemic: Effects of stay-at-home policies, social distancing behavior, and social resources', *Psychiatry Research*, 293, p. 113419.

McDonald, R. I., Yi Chai, H. and Newell, B. (2015), 'Personal experience and the "psychological distance" of climate change: An integrative review', *Journal of Environmental Psychology*, 44, pp. 109–18.

McPherson, K. E., McAloney-Kocaman, K., McGlinchey, E., Faeth, P. and Armour, C. (2021), 'Longitudinal analysis of the UK COVID-19 Psychological Wellbeing Study: Trajectories of anxiety, depression and COVID-19-related stress symptomology', *Psychiatry Research*, 304, p. 114138.

Melodia, F., Canale, N. and Griffiths, M. D. (2020), 'The role of avoidance coping and escape motives in problematic online gaming: A systematic literature review', *International Journal of Mental Health and Addiction*, 20, pp. 996–1022 https://doi.org/10.1007/s11469-020-00422-w.

Michaelson, J., Mahony, S. and Schifferes, J. (2012), *Measuring Well-Being: A Guide for Practitioners*, London: New Economics Foundation.

Middleton, V. T. and Lickorish, L. J. (2007), *British Tourism: The Remarkable Story of Growth*, London: Routledge.

National Trust (2019), *2019 Handbook*, London: Wyndeham Group.

National Trust (2020), *National Trust Annual Report 2019/20*, Swindon: National Trust, https://gat04-live-1517c8a4486c41609369c68f30c8-aa81074.divio-media.org/filer_public/a2/39/a2399301-f1d8-4396-a69e-a368dd3b7b56/rvr-w1-2-3.pdf. Accessed 25 March 2023.

O'Connor, R. C., Wetherall, K., Cleare, S., McClelland, H., Melson, A. J., Niedzwiedz, C. L., O'Carroll, R. E., O'Connor, D. B., Platt, S., Scowcroft, E. and Watson, B. (2021), 'Mental health and well-being during the COVID-19 pandemic: Longitudinal analyses of adults in the UK COVID-19 Mental Health & Wellbeing study', *The British Journal of Psychiatry*, 218:6, pp. 326–33.

Office of National Statistics (2020), 'Coronavirus and the social impacts on Great Britain: 19 June 2020', https://b.3cdn.net/nefoundation/8d92cf44e70b3d16e6_rgm6bpd3i.pdf; https://www.ons.gov.uk/peoplepopulationandcommunity/healthandsocialcare/healthandwellbeing/bulletins/coronavirusandthesocialimpactsongreatbritain/19june2020. Accessed 25 March 2023.

Pine, J. and Gilmore, J. (1998), 'Welcome to the experience economy', *Harvard Business Review*, July–August, pp. 97–105.

Ponsignon, F., Lunardo, R. and Michrafy, M. (2021), 'Why are international visitors more satisfied with the tourism experience? The role of hedonic value, escapism, and psychic distance', *Journal of Travel Research*, 60:8, pp. 1771–86.

Radder, L., Han, X. and Hou, Y. (2011), 'An integrated evaluation of the heritage museum visit: A disconfirmation approach', *International Journal of Management Cases*, 13:3, pp. 315–26.

Reynolds, N. (2006), 'Ruinous expense of stopping Corfe Castle from crumbling', *The Daily Telegraph*, 23 August, https://www.telegraph.co.uk/news/1526996/Ruinous-expense-of-stopping-Corfe-Castle-from-crumbling.html. Accessed 25 March 2023.

Rojek, C. (1997), 'Indexing, dragging and the social construction of tourist sights', in C. Rojek and J. Urry (eds), *Touring Cultures. Transformations of Travel and Theory*, London: Routledge, pp. 52–74.

Scarpi, D. and Raggiotto, F. (2023), 'A construal level view of contemporary heritage tourism', *Tourism Management*, 94, p. 104648.

Seaton, A. V. (2002), 'Tourism as metempsychosis and metensomatosis: The personae of eternal recurrence', in G. M. S. Dann (ed.), *The Tourist as a Metaphor of the Social World*, Oxon: CABI, pp. 135–68.

Smith, M. (2003), 'Holistic holidays: Tourism and the reconciliation of body, mind and spirit', *Tourism Recreation Research*, 28:1, pp. 103–08.

Sofaer, J., Davenport, B., Sørensen, M. L. S., Gallou, E. and Uzzell, D. (2021), 'Heritage sites, value and wellbeing: Learning from the COVID-19 pandemic in England', *International Journal of Heritage Studies*, 27:11, pp. 1117–32.

Spender, S. (1974), *Love-Hate Relations: A Study of Anglo-American Sensibilities*, London: Hamish Hamilton.

Suntikul, W. and Jachna, T. (2016), 'Profiling the heritage experience in Macao's historic center', *International Journal of Tourism Research*, 18, pp. 308–18.

Thurley, S. (2013), *The Men from the Ministry: How Britain Saved Its Heritage*, London and New Haven, CT: Yale University Press.

Trope, Y. and Liberman, N. (2010), 'Construal-level theory of psychological distance', *Psychological Review*, 117, pp. 440–63.

Trunfio, M., Lucia, M. D., Campana, S. and Magnelli, A. (2022), 'Innovating the cultural heritage museum service model through virtual reality and augmented reality: The effects on the overall visitor experience and satisfaction', *Journal of Heritage Tourism*, 17:1, pp. 1–19.

Tull, M. T., Edmonds, K. A., Scamaldo, K. M., Richmond, J. R., Rose, J. P. and Gratz, K. L. (2020), 'Psychological outcomes associated with stay-at-home orders and the perceived impact of COVID-19 on daily life', *Psychiatry Research*, 289, pp. 113098–106.

Urry, J. (1990), *The Tourist Gaze*, London: Sage.

Urry, J. (1996), 'How societies remember the past', in S. MacDonald and G. Fyfe (eds), *Theorizing the Museum: Representing Identity and Diversity in a Changing World*, Oxford: Blackwell, pp. 45–68.

Vorderer, P. (1996), 'Rezeptionsmotivation: Warum nutzen Rezipienten mediale Unterhaltungsangebote?' *Publizistik*, 41:3, pp. 310–26.

Walsh, K. (1992), *The Representation of the Past: Museums and Heritage in the Post-Modern World*, London: Routledge.

White, R. (2014), 'Time travel: Australian tourists and Britain's past', *Portal: Journal of Multidisciplinary International Studies*, 11:1, pp. 1–25.

Wilson, A. (2020), 'National Trust begins phased reopening of gardens and parklands', *The Guardian*, 28 May, https://www.theguardian.com/travel/2020/may/28/national-trust-begins-phased-reopening-of-gardens-and-parklands. Accessed 25 March 2023.

Wilson, R. and Mackley, A. (2000), *Creating Paradise: The Building of the English Country House, 1660–1880*, London: Hambledon and London.

Wong, J. C., Yang, J. Z. and Liu, Z. (2022), 'It's the thoughts that count: How psychological distance and affect heuristic influence support for aid response measures during the COVID-19 pandemic', *Health Communication*, 38:12, pp. 2702–10, https://doi.org/10.1080/10410236.2022.2109394.

3

Ritualization of 'Distance' in Christian Liturgy during the Plague

Piotr Roszak and Piotr Paweł Orłowski

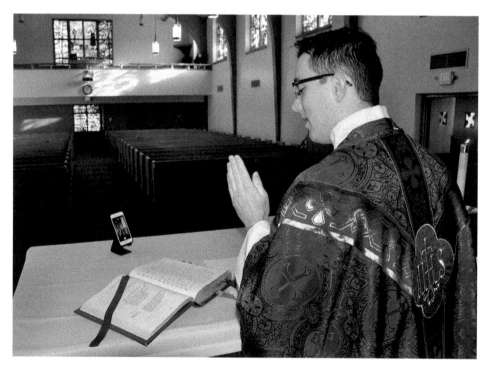

FIGURE 3.1: The streaming of a holy mass during the COVID-19 pandemic. Courtesy of https://media.defense.gov/ Ⓢ.

Plague provides an opportunity to verify certain rituals that have existed up until now and to consider the emergence of new ones that have created the circumstances of the pandemic. The images of religious rites that appeared in media reporting on the pandemic primarily exposed the spatial changes that were expressed in keeping distance between the faithful. The assigned and distant places that people could take up in churches created an unnatural distance for the liturgy, which seemed to undermine the spoken words about gathering, community and closeness of the faithful with Christ and with one another. Caution and health concerns collided with the essence of liturgical action, which emphasizes the joint performance of activities (*leiton ergon*), and the Church itself is defined as a holy convocation (*kahal Jahve*) and gathering into one.

Nevertheless, this liturgical distance during the time of the plague, which sanctioned 'social distance', including the restrictions – for instance, on greeting, which was dealt with in many ways (with elbow, thumb, a bow, etc.) – as a way of overcoming the transmission of the virus, must be part of a wider trend (Katila et al. 2020). This necessitated the search for new forms of engagement in shared experiences or emotions. In a sense, this is an expected reaction because the history of liturgy is woven with the emergence and integration of new rites that form an organic totality, so the changes are not only sectoral but affect the whole (Bell 1989). Celebrations are not immutable forms of cultic behaviour but are subject to actualizations and reinterpretations. Physical distance began to be contrasted with spiritual closeness, which, incidentally, somehow revealed many of the subconscious anthropological assumptions of the liturgy (largely Platonic, depreciating the body and focusing on spiritual experience). The ritual responses to plagues in the history of liturgy show this perfectly: the emergence of new rites, as well as the modification of existing ones.

In this respect, the presence of rituals and their significance for Christian gatherings are presented first, then following this, the most important COVID-related changes within the liturgy in 2020–21 in order to finally focus on the various forms of distance that the pandemic introduced into the celebrations. The starting point for the analysis will be some images depicting the implemented social distance and the ways of its ritualization, especially taking into account the redefinition of certain ritual behaviours or customs, which, to the surprise of many, have returned to the liturgy years after being discontinued (e.g. the use of gloves), though not in the same form as earlier. Framing distance in this way, from a socio-theological perspective, provokes questions about deeper transformations for Christian piety. The tension that has appeared between the closeness of God declared in prayers and celebrations and fellow believers among themselves, as well as the physical barriers introduced by distance, prompts observation of the impact this will have on the experience of the liturgy after the plague.

Ritual and its significance for religious life

It is relevant to pay attention to the importance of rituals in experiencing reality before moving on to describing the ways of coping with the experience of restrictions that were introduced to the liturgy during the pandemic. This significance is revealed with exceptional force, especially in border situations, as a manifestation of coping; that is to say, as a way of experiencing difficulties in a beneficial way, which is typical of religiosity as well as in other anthropological contexts (Oviedo 2019). The human is a ritual being because rite as a 'repeatable activity reflecting meaning' signifies entering into an essential relationship with the world. In this sense, it constitutes a kind of language that is close to a symbolic language, due to which a certain way of human habitation in the world is being marked. Things are not ritualized for no reason but are instead perpetuated through repeatable gestures and actions that translate into human identity. The appearance of rituals in everyday life consists not only of the discovery of simple rules for the consequences of different behaviours (what we do and how we do it in a certain order, e.g. getting up every morning) but in a strong sense, it signifies a person's focus on what cannot be omitted.

Therefore, in this context, this focus is actually referred to as 'ritual memory', which wants to open up to the future rather than preserve the past so that it will not be forgotten too quickly. Rituals not only aim to salvage detailed issues from past history but also to apply the old ones to the current situation. This is perhaps best seen in liturgical rituals, such as the Haggadah used in Passover when the story of the liberation from Egypt is told (Griffiths 2021: 13) or in Christmas rituals in Christian culture (e.g. in Poland). Nonetheless, repeatable symbolic activity acquires meaning through narration and a certain analogy; however, there is often a change in the importance of the activities despite the duration of the external ritual. This phenomenon was described by Welte, referring to the lack of meaning (*umwesen*), which introduces a dichotomy between the external and internal and breaks the thread connecting them (Welte 1952). Empty rituals appear, whose significance does not convince those who fulfil and observe them. It might be noted that distance in the liturgy is also in danger of becoming ritualized in this sense; it will be maintained as a repeatable activity even after the threats have ceased.

Hence, leaving the possible atrophies of ritual aside, yet another of its functions in the liturgical context was revealed during the pandemic – relevant to the topic about distance that we are dealing with here – one that becomes a stabilizer of meanings that expresses ways of perceiving and speaking about the world. Due to the repetition of ritual gestures, settling is achieved – that is, regaining control over certain areas of life that were shaken by the pandemic. In the face of fear of infection, the ritualization of distance leaves a kind of message about the possibility of getting this situation under control (Marcus and McCullough 2021). It does not have to do with eliminating particular rituals, but changing, modifying or transforming them. Other rites that correct the ritual serve this purpose, providing a new form of meaning and saving the whole ritual system, where one element suffers from semantic undermining.

Beyond the liturgical context, Legare highlighted the emerging COVID rituals that began to address new social challenges. As with certain social conventions, rituals are not arbitrary but reveal the subjects' state of mind and perform critical functions in a given situation. In addition, their important role is to express solidarity within the community by allowing communities to express their shared goals and values. In other words, ritual behaviours reproduce the semantic common field by revealing what is protected. A ritual is thus a form of bonding the community together by watching over the expressions of its beliefs (Czachesz 2017: 101). This is particularly relevant to celebration because the Christian liturgy is a ritual system in which the theological presupposition is being embodied.

In an epistemological context, however, Flanagan draws attention to an essential feature of the rite that implicitly acknowledges apophaticism, which is overcome by ritualization. The inability to know reality in full does not end with silence but in an attempt to manifest the discovered truth, even if it is only partial. In this regard, within the Christian liturgy, particularly the Eucharist, it is worth noting the ritual attempt to manage the absence of Christ, who, through transubstantiation, is being recovered in a visible form. The epiclesis, the ritual repetition of the words of Christ from the Last Supper, accomplishes a transformation involving the participants because an 'extraordinary exchange' takes place: the fruit of the work of the hands, which is brought to the celebration and symbolized in bread, becomes the substance of the sacrament. This shows that the ritual not only creates the possibility of grasping the mystery that transcends but is also a resource of connection through which healing is experienced (Imber-Black and Roberts 1998).

In this respect, it is worth noting the interesting study by Belcher on how new rites appear in an already-formed system, as a ritualized body does not seem to enable changes (Belcher 2019). This is well exemplified in the rituals of folk piety, which complemented official ritualization in the era of plagues, such as the processions of flagellants wandering around Europe during the Black Death period (1348–50) (Gobel 2017). This ritualization does not occur without a certain theological background; in the case of the flagellants, the wrath of God was overcome by an act of repentance, which drew attention to questions about God's will, which, after all, were undertaken by the nominalists of that time in the discussions defeating Thomistic intellectualism. Because people are unable to find an explanation for the plague in the existing ritual experience, which emphasizes the ordering of the world and the care of the Divine Providence, new rituals are being prepared by a theology that is strongly based on voluntarism. Due to the fact that God wants the plague, such a ritual behaviour thus becomes the only effective method that could propitiate the will of the angry creator. This can be done by a person undertaking severe penance. Regarding the coronavirus pandemic, certain ritual behaviours were certainly prepared by theological reflections that attempted to interpret the experience of suffering.

This, however, raises broader questions about how reference to the symbolic language introduced into the liturgy is made. Gomez Rincon distinguishes three features: (1) the symbol complements the lack of literal language by revealing relationships and similarities that in fact cannot be equated, but the differences are preserved (paternity of God and human), and it is an attempt to describe the indescribable Transcendence, lest it becomes an idol, (2) creating a new relationship to the divine – hence the symbol has the function of enabling an encounter with the Thou, and not merely a discursive one and (3) discovering the meaning of the world since symbols establish the order of the world, which is then featured (Gomez Rincon 2020: 186–89).

Meanwhile, considerations of the role of rituals fall within the logic of the liturgy. Liturgy is not a set of texts or descriptions of an abstract reality, a kind of sacred game, but a system of practice and the very actions expressed through rituals (Gschwandtner 2021). Contemporary liturgical theology thus distinguishes between *theologia prima* – the liturgy itself as a cultic activity, and *theologia secunda*, that is, everything that emerges from the liturgy and is described by words. Diversity in accessing these experiences is possible in such a lived system, and ritual differentiation allows for the capture of key contrasts or ambivalences in the different behaviours of individuals. Such is the case with the relations of the participants in the liturgy, among which a tension appears between the expression of unity (all participants in the liturgy are one community – one body) and the discernible difference between those who form this community. This opens up interpretative possibilities for ritual behaviour that must consider both poles; by avoiding reductionist explanations, they allow for a symbolic approach.

In order to unite the Eucharist with daily life, the post-conciliar reform brought it close to an embodied gesture or posture, and this was also done throughout the pandemic; otherwise, there could be a risk of alienation. The same applied to the Eucharist and the daily meal: there was a strong connection between the two but also a visible difference (what St. Paul reminded the Corinthians in his letter to them). Likewise, with distance, which was an everyday occurrence at the time of COVID-19, there could be no breaking of this experience in the liturgy, but there was a need to ritualize it and show its meaning in a broader theological context.

Plague and changes in liturgy: What new changes has the COVID-19 pandemic brought?

The appearance of the coronavirus introduced turbulence into the liturgical life of communities, which were not able to celebrate the liturgy at all (it was suspended) or suffered significant restrictions; however, it also provoked a specific response: rejection or adaptation. Not all responses were ritualistic in nature, which was referred to earlier. However, it is worth mentioning here the specific type of homily or security measures related to the counting of the faithful (e.g. gates where the faithful were being counted or candies distributed in line with the admissible number of participants in the liturgy), the use of holy water from dispensers so as not to touch the same container of water or baptism carried out in some Christian communities in the United States with a garden hose to avoid contact between the minister and the recipient of the sacrament (Dallas 2020). These are similarly important because they show the broader changes taking place.

From a historical perspective, what were the ritualizations of earlier plagues? It is interesting to pay attention to the elements that the pandemic brought with it in terms of liturgy and architecture. In St. John's Cathedral in Toruń, the image of the 'Black Death' appears, painted in such a way as to make people leaving the sanctuary aware of the victims of the pandemic as an experience of God's punishment (in the medieval mentality, plagues were a symbol of the coming of antichrist), but also new liturgical forms, such as the singing of supplications appeared earlier in the patristic period (McCormick 2021). This term covers a song of supplication for the pandemic to end, asking for God's mercy on his people and preserving them from disasters. This was sung at special moments in the history of Polish Catholicism and was reinstated during COVID-19 throughout services and at the end of the Eucharist. Penitential processions (in Rome with the cross) were, in the past, an expression of a request for atonement and release, to which there has been a return, for example, during the penitential service celebrated by Pope Francis at the empty St. Peter's Square, which, unlike those of previous eras, highlighted other theological themes, such as fraternity and solidarity, not contradicting traditional ones, but definitely putting those in the shade.

In ancient liturgical traditions, numerous votive masses appeared, the motive of which included a request to remain healthy while experiencing *tribulationes*. Special collections of sermons also arose, such as the four themes from the 'Homily of Toledo', which illustrate the effects of plague on religiosity. These called for repentance and revision of life, trust in God and prayer with the 'lamentations' as a specific form of relationship with God in the midst of troubles. It is clear that the new forms of response to the pandemic within the liturgy were a manifestation of disillusionment with the institutions, altering the collective imagination by consolidating certain shared experiences.

Pontifical versus COVID gloves: 'Tactile' distance

During the COVID-19 pandemic, some Christian churches returned to giving Holy Communion with gloves, which had a practical function in view of the threat of transmission of the virus; they were supposed to protect the celebrant and ensure that the sacrament was received safely. This behaviour was not new to the Christian tradition but brought a significant change to its semantic sphere, thus giving the old ritual a new context.

Before the reform of the Second Vatican Council, gloves (Latin *chirothecæ* or *manicæ*) were used by bishops and the Pope during solemn liturgies, especially at Mass. The tradition began in the eleventh century, and permission to use gloves was a privilege granted by the Pope to bishops and abbots. They were initially made of linen, and then from the twelfth century silk, and they were decorated with special embroideries, medals and precious stones. The latter disappeared at the end of the Middle Ages, leaving room only for cloth gloves.[1] The decorations were references to the Eucharist, and their colour expressed a given liturgical period, that is Lent, Christmas, Ordinary Time, etc. (Perrin and Vasco 1999). When bishops celebrated the Eucharist, they used gloves from the beginning until they went to the altar during the offering and then took them off and put them back on again for the rite of the pontifical blessing at the end.

The use of gloves was not dictated by practical reasons, such as keeping the hands warm on frosty days, but was intended to express the concern for moral chastity with which the celebrant proceeds to celebrate the great mysteries. The symbolic meaning is explained in the prayer uttered by the bishop at the moment of putting on the gloves, just after having put on the dalmatics. It recalls a situation in the life of patriarch Jacob, who covered himself with goatskins to resemble Esau and receive his father's blessing (cf. Gen. 27:16 nn.). The gloves on the bishop's hands thus signified a request for the blessing of God, to whom he is accountable for those entrusted to his care. It is thereby an indication of the purity of intentions with which the consecrated person acts in the service of the people of God. There is no hygienic rationale here, though no doubt it brings such as well. This is, in fact, typical of the Thomistic approach, in which religiosity is beneficial to nature since grace is granted to it.

In modern times, following liturgical changes that have taken place, gloves are no longer part of the pontifical vestments. It is, however, interesting to note the transformation from secular use, from which it passed into liturgy in the eleventh century, after being used during the last pandemic. In ecclesiastical ordinances, for instance, in Italy on 7 May 2020, this was recommended:

> The distribution of Communion will take place after the celebrant and the possible extraordinary minister have taken care of the hygiene of their hands and worn disposable gloves; the same person – wearing the mask, taking care to cover their nose and mouth and maintaining an adequate safety distance – takes care to offer the host without coming into contact with the hands of the faithful.
>
> (Catholic Church)

Gloves made of latex or other materials appear frequently with regard to giving Holy Communion in other denominations as well, whether in churches or during celebrations outside, such as those held in a parking lot.[2] This stirred up a lot of controversy and strong reactions that emphasized changes in the essence of the sign and the desacralization of the sacrament: after the consecration, every particle is cared for, but it is difficult to do that with gloves on. Furthermore, the gloves create distance between the celebrant and Christ present in the Eucharistic species. It deprives the liturgy of the essential experience of 'touch' that appears and is symbolized in the liturgical action in many different ways.

Face mask – 'visual' distance

Even though it was used on a daily basis in times of the pandemic, the appearance of the face mask with regard to the liturgy created yet another type of distance between the people participating in the rite. It is a distance created not for the sense of touch (like gloves) but for the eyes, thus making it difficult to build communities.

In order to break this specific distance, the mask began to be introduced into many liturgical performances, starting with the motifs of Christmas cribs in which the characters from the Gospels who assist in the birth of Christ wear face masks (as Mary and Joseph or the three kings). At times, the depictions of Christ on the Cross also had a mask on His face to show solidarity with the people. This was, however, definitely different from that adopted in the Christian liturgy, although with varied lengths of application (e.g. in the Mozarabic and Roman Rite), as the covering of the cross and altars, which are unveiled on Good Friday, during the last period of Lent.

Ritualization of distance and its forms in regard to the Christian liturgy

It is worth noting that many studies on the impact of social distancing on the life of Christian communities most often consider the scenario of suspending celebrations altogether and broadcasting them online (Adegboyega et al. 2021). Attention is paid to the changes introduced by virtual celebrations, with a focus on whether they lead to the same spiritual fruits as when experienced in the church directly or whether they bring consolation or build bonds and social capital; however, few consider the importance of distance and restrictions with regard to the liturgy already celebrated. This provokes questions about why it is worth coming to the church, rather than continuing to attend via a screen. In trying to understand people's choices, some have turned to game theory (Huang 2022), showing the rationale for choosing a certain risk over a certain benefit. A number of distance-shortening initiatives, such as celebrations in cars (Chow 2020), in the open air and so on, can attest to the important form of overcoming virtual participation.

However, we will take other forms of ritualization of distance into consideration, which can be seen in the in-person celebrations that have already taken place. The experience of participating in a ritual, as Émile Durkheim noted, allows for a sort of emotional contagion that he called 'collective effervescence'. Ritualization will thus mean the process of giving meaning to the distance that has emerged as a result of the plague and is gaining new meaning: it provokes compensatory behaviour, thanks to which the sense of liturgical celebration will be preserved.

Distance among the faithful

Distance in churches was introduced in many ways. In some cases, the faithful were free to take up space; in others, it was suggested that they occupy only every second bench, with tape being used to mark the spaces to be excluded from use; others returned to assigning specific places, but keeping social distance. Although the layout of the celebration has always been subject to changes, it was built on the basis of a structure excluding the presbytery from the place for the people; it was not for isolation, but rather a demonstration of the hierarchy.

How has there been an attempt to break this experience of physical distance and ritual behaviour, which contradicts the essence of liturgical gathering? Many of the gestures are intended to maintain the bond between the faithful, starting with passing the sign of peace with a directed gaze and bow. However, many have become accustomed to showing unity with others through touch gestures, such as a kiss of peace or a handshake. In the medieval liturgy, there was a specific way of communicating peace, which was through the so-called pax (Nadolski 2006), which were small rectangular or oval plates with a handle that the celebrants passed to each other. These contained ornaments referring mainly to the Passion of Christ. Later on, relics began to be placed in them, which were made available for the faithful to kiss and kept in the sacristies covered by a coloured veil.

Nowadays, one speaks of a triple mode of spatial relation, which is determined by the criterion of the dominance of a certain sense. On the one hand, it concerns 'perceiving', which is about noticing something in the scenery, while on the other, 'conceiving', which regards a cognitive apprehension and identification of a place and a 'live' experience, where the bodily presence leads to the establishment of a relationship (Daelemans 2020). This, in turn, leads to a relational recognition of 'sacrum' (Roszak 2020).

The distance required during the pandemic affected the relations between the celebrant and the altar servers who do not approach the altar, leaving all the paraments previously prepared. That way, there is no *lavabo* gesture, which the minister performs himself (and sometimes uses antibacterial gel instead of water). One is left with the impression of the celebrant being physically alone, even though the concelebrants still surround the altar.

The procession of the faithful wanting to receive Holy Communion is what helps break the distance. Despite keeping their distance from each other and wearing masks, the faithful approach the altar, the centre that connects them to each other. Nonetheless, even here, they come across signs that emphasize the dialectics of this distance, because, after all, communion means closeness, whereas distance contradicts it – an example of this is a praxis from the cathedral in Cologne, Germany, where the very moment of receiving Holy Communion took place under a pane of plexiglass.

Liturgical philosophy of distance: Tension overcome

The ritual behaviours described earlier, which refer to distance in liturgy, serve to highlight an issue that is inherent in the nature of celebration. It refers to past events, which it makes present through *anamensis*. This is expressed by the Latin terms used to describe the mysteries celebrated, such as *repraesentatio* and frequent references to the liturgical 'today'. Time distance is the matter of liturgical action, which is overcome by reference, not to a linear but a participatory arrangement of time. This means that – according to a certain philosophy behind the Christian rite – the liturgy does not distance itself from its source each year, but establishes a direct relationship to the mystery through participation in it. Therefore, it is not about concealing the distance or blurring the differences: distance brings awareness about a certain equality to that which is being exercised, regardless of the times in which someone is living. This is expressed, according to Pickstock, in how the liturgy treats the meanings of the words that are being used: they are not terms devoid of any relation to what they stand for (ambiguous sense) nor the same (unambiguous), but they are analogous in nature. What the terms mean is accomplished in a real though sacramental way (Pickstock 1998). Otherwise, as

Pickstock notes, we would be dealing with a semantic rupture that leads to a kind of intellectual necrophilia. Then again, liturgy is about a live experience and not a nostalgic recollection of distant events.

There is yet a different kind of distance that has emerged at the time of the plague, associated with the so-called tele-liturgy broadcast by the media and described by some as a new mutation of the old Docetism, only this time of a liturgical nature. As such, while defending the deity of Christ, Docetism negated His corporeality and the realism of His suffering on the cross, thus introducing a vision of Christ as the disembodied Messiah. This translated into coping with distance by accepting it and trying to build the liturgy in isolation from the bodily reception of the sacraments as a matter of principle (rather than as a temporary experience for the duration of epidemiological restrictions).

The distance between the faithful, their origins, wealth and education is inscribed by the liturgy in the equality of all believers and refers to the spatial distance of the way towards the source symbolized by the altar. The path to it is an expression of the faithful drawing closer to one another as they move towards Christ. Thus, it can be seen that the point is not to blur differences on a dialectical basis and remove paradoxical tension but to maintain a paradox (distant but close) that is reconcilable at a higher level of interpretation. Simultaneously, the 'difference' – a theme present in postmodern philosophy – is not dissolved, but is consistent with the Trinitarian dogma, which maintains the oneness of God with the diversity of the persons of the Trinity, thus becoming the path to unity.

Theological challenges in the time of plague

It is worth taking up some other theological questions caused by the emergence of distance in experiencing liturgy. Introducing a semantic dissonance (the sign ceases to signify the content it expresses) disturbs the hitherto scheme and, at the same time, allows one to see new dimensions. Gathering all the disciples of Christ together, by definition, means destroying the distance ('wall') that existed before coming to faith. In line with this, St. Paul points to the fact that Christ came to overcome the distance between Jews and other nations, between slaves and the free, women and men (cf. Gal. 3:28). Keeping distance and ritualizing it seem to theologically challenge the basic principles of the liturgy. Let us focus on three aspects.

Sacrament of relationship: Does distance still express fraternity?

The first aspect concerns the definition of liturgy from the perspective of the relationships it establishes, which, on the one hand, consists of an ongoing relationship with God, and on the other, a relationship between the participants. Therefore, the Eucharist as building the Church can be seen as a kind of sacrament of relationships: it introduces relationships and shapes them through love, where Christ's love is its model. During the pandemic, an attempt to overcome spatial distance with visual contact could be observed, which stems from the concern that the relationship should be based on a sense (in this case, eyesight) and not just an idea. The category of relationships was of exceptional importance as early as Aristotle, who defined it as being directed towards the other, to something. It is not strictly 'something' in being, but expresses its dynamics in creating bonds. In this sense, the Christian liturgy emphasizes the coherence between participation in the celebration and the bond, and hence fraternity between the participants in the liturgy. This typically Christian approach – the emphasis on relationships, both in the dimension of Trinitarian theology and existence – is one of the criteria used today for evaluating what is authentically human, and this is highlighted, for example, by Donati's relational sociology (Donati and Maspero 2021). In the reality of the pandemic, distance does not make relationships impossible, but creates a new context for the very existence of distance, as Chillon notes, which is a condition for a relationship with another, and not its cancellation (Chillon 2016: 33). The other person can only be regarded from a certain distance.

Distance as a limitation and an opportunity

Attention is also drawn to the fact that a pandemic creates an experience of liminality and, therefore, a certain threshold transition from one cycle to another. It is about the triple structure indicated by Turner, who talks about the pre-liminal and post-liminal, as well as the experience of the transition itself. Nobody doubts that the plague is not a permanent condition and that the *communitas* that are being formed in the recovery from the pandemic will be a challenge to reintegrate the community. Its reconstruction will involve a return to the essence of the liturgy and a new context or experience. In the times of Roman domestic worship, the appearance of plagues caused a verification of worship, the removal of new deities, and the introduction of new sacrificial customs (Cianca 2018: 61).

The post-pandemic ritual-liturgical practice will not be the same as it was before. The community can reflect on the use of space beforehand because the plague teaches a certain equality; it does not discriminate or affect, for example, only the wicked (Scott 2020). What follows is what some call heterotopia, a space of contrast. It is about the experience of inclusiveness that the plague triggers; therefore, overcoming the distance will involve a different understanding of space. This will involve inviting people to defeat barriers and live the promise; participation in the ritual equalizes participants who remain vulnerable to the same degree.

Simultaneously, there is talk about the ritualization of hygiene in the post-pandemic time, which may be significant, for example, by limiting singing during the liturgy (and this in itself has an important ritual dimension) and imposing restrictions on contact, but also in terms of being a church after the pandemic.

One can speak, therefore, of the unexpected consequences of social distancing in liturgical gatherings, which are observed not only by theologians but also by psychologists. The latter divide the effects into positive ones, such as technological innovations in communicating a message relevant to the community, and into negative ones, like the decline of cohesion, the social capital of communities, identity imbalance established by a long tradition, and practices specific to these denominations, especially the liturgy. Many studies emphasize the psychological damage to believers who did not meet during the pandemic, thus making certain spiritual and mental problems worse (such as depression, anxiety, etc.).

Distance versus 'watching' the liturgy

Participation in the so-called tele-liturgy (Barnard et al. 2014), thus, observing the celebration virtually from home, was another form of experiencing distance during the pandemic. In times of the dominance of a specific eye-centrism, that is, the domination of only seeing and perceiving, rather than conceiving and experiencing – live (three stages in the perception of architecture according to Lefebvre) participation at a distance discloses itself as inadequate and reveals deeper problems. Following a broadcast image is not the same as participating in the celebration; as Izquierdo notes, it is about grasping that something is happening during the liturgy in which one partakes (Izquierdo 2020). It is not enough to be informed about it.

The ritualization of distance by viewing through the media, which would make churches unnecessary, even reinforced by the forms and canon of behaviour during such broadcasts (which have been undertaken by religious communities and prepared for the faithful in some countries) is so far-reaching that it loses the sense of the liturgy. For the essence is the gathering into one around the altar, and thus leaving the house to be at the liturgy (which, throughout history, also took on a ritualistic nature by saying goodbye to household members, from clothing to the very way of reaching places of worship). Leaving daily duties for the purpose of going to a holy place, and hence approaching the sacred, is connected to experiencing the liturgy, which cannot be reduced to a simple communication process because it involves the whole person. In this context, the liturgical value of 'touch' or closeness becomes understandable (e.g. rites of blessings with outstretched hands over the faithful). Therefore, new rituals will have to incorporate the sense of liturgical action (granting grace) with new opportunities for participation, thanks to the new means of communication. At the time of the pandemic, the virtual distance in many countries was already supplemented by individual visits to churches and private prayers of the faithful during different times of the day. The core message, however, is for the community to discover the value of the liturgy, which is not something additional but a certain way of life.

Conclusion – Is a new ritualistic piety being born? How the plague is changing the experience of religiosity

The described changes in the Christian liturgy caused by COVID-19 bring variations in the ritual behaviour of believers, but they also shape a new piety. The experience of a specific 'fasting', consisting of living some distance from another person, leads to the realization of the value of closeness, which becomes rediscovered with all its symbolic baggage. This is appropriate for the post-liminal state when one returns to the essence, which cannot be lost in the course of history. The ritualization of hygienic behaviour will have to collide with the theological basis: it is an opportunity for new rituals to represent renewal, rather than a mere repetition of earlier behaviours (Tytarenko and Bogachevska 2021). Rituals rooted in reality have always been perceived as a means of changing the state of affairs.

At the same time, however, the changes affect the paradigm shift within piety (Blázquez 2021). The pandemic has caused a change in piety; in fact, the first signs of it have already been seen by some, where piety ceases to be identified with 'place' and begins to be dominated by 'relationship'. Paradoxically, this turns out to be closer to the classical understanding of *devotio*, which did not merely rely on the performance of certain acts labelled as religious, but on binding the human to the ultimate goal.

NOTES

1. https://asociacionliturgicamagnificat.blogspot.com/2016/10/los-ornamentos-e-insignias-de-los.html. Accessed 20 October 2023.
2. https://www.inquirer.com/health/coronavirus/coronavirus-covid19-philadelphia-pennsylvania-new-jersey-christianity-judaism-sunday-worship-20200315.html. Accessed 9 July 2023.

REFERENCES

Adegboyega, A., Boddie, S., Dorvie, H., Bolaji, B., Adedoyin, C. and Moore, S. E. (2021), 'Social distance impact on church gatherings: Socio-behavioral implications', *Journal of Human Behavior in the Social Environment*, 31:1–4, pp. 221–34.

Barnard, M., Cilliers, J. and Wepener, C. (2014), *Worship in the Network Culture: Liturgical Ritual Studies. Fields and Methods, Concepts and Metaphors, Liturgia Condenda 28*, Leuven: Peeters.

Belcher, K. (2019), 'Ritual systems, ritualized bodies, and the laws of liturgical development', *Studia Liturgica*, 49:1, pp. 89–110.

Bell, C. (1989), 'Ritual, change, and changing rituals', *Worship*, 63, pp. 31–41.

Blázquez, N. (2021), 'Covid-19 y pastoral liturgica', *Studium*, 61:1, pp. 37–74.

Catholic Church (2020), *The Protocol*, art. 3.4, https://www.chiesacattolica.it/dal-18-maggio-celebrazioni-con-il-popolo/. Accessed 03 June 2024.

Chillon, J. M. (2016), *El pensar y la distancia. Hacia una comprension de la critica como filosofia*, Salamanca: Sigueme.

Chow, A. R. (2020), 'Come as you are in the family car. Drive-in church services are taking off during the coronavirus pandemic', *Time*, 28 March, https://time.com/5811387/drive-in-church-coronavirus. Accessed 23 April 2023.

Cianca, J. (2018), *Sacred Ritual, Profane Space: The Roman House as Early Christian Meeting Place*, Montreal: McGill-Queen's University Press.

Czachesz, I. (2017), *Cognitive Science and the New Testament: A New Approach to Early Christian Research*, Oxford: OPU.

Daelemans, B. (2020), 'Healing space: The synaesthetic quality of church architecture', *Religions*, 11, p. 635, https://doi.org/10.3390/rel11120635.

Dallas, K. (2020), 'How the pandemic is reshaping baptism rituals in churches across the country', *DeseretNews*, 2 June, https://www.deseret.com/indepth/2020/6/1/21272505/coronavirus-church-closures-baptism-ritual-pandemic-pastor-new-jersey-texas-illinois-covid-19. Accessed 23 April 2023.

Donati, P. and Maspero, G. (2021), *Dopo la pandemia. Rigenerare la società con le relazioni*, Roma: Città Nuova.

Gobel, E. (2017), 'Liturgical processions in the Black Death', *The Hilltop Review*, 9:2, art. 5.

Gomez Rincon, C. (2020), *Racionalidad y trascendencia. Investigaciones en epistemología de la religión*, Santander: Sal Terrae.

Griffiths, A. (2021), *Identity and Ritual*, Oxford: SLG Press.

Gschwandtner, C. M. (2021), 'Is liturgy ludic? Distinguishing between the phenomena of play and ritual', *Religions*, 12:4, art. 232.

Huang, Y. and Zhu, Q. (2022), 'Game-theoretic frameworks for epidemic spreading and human decision-making: A review', *Dynamic Games and Applications*, 12, pp. 7–48.

Imber-Black, E. and Roberts, J. (1998), *Rituals for Our Times: Celebrating, Healing and Changing Our Lives and Our Relationships*, Northvale: Jason Aronson.

Izquierdo, C. (2020), 'Covid-19 z perspektywy chrześcijańskiej', *Warszawskie Studia Teologiczne*, 33:2, pp. 26–41.

Katila J., Gan, Y. and Goodwin, M. H. (2020), 'Interaction rituals and "social distancing": New haptic trajectories and touching from a distance in the time of COVID-19', *Discourse Studies*, 22:4, pp. 418–40.

Marcus, Z. J. and McCullough, M. E. (2021), 'Does religion make people more self-controlled? A review of research from the lab and life', *Current Opinion in Psychology*, 40, pp. 167–70.

McCormick, M. (2021), 'Gregory of Tours on sixth-century plague and other epidemics', *Speculum*, 96:1, pp. 38–96.

Nadolski, B. (2006), *Leksykon liturgii*, Poznań: Wydawnictwo Pallottinum.

Oviedo, L. (2019), 'Meaning and religion: Exploring mutual implications', *Scientia et Fides*, 7:1, pp. 25–46.

Pentin, E. (2020), 'Public masses resume in Italy, but not without controversy', *National Catholic Register*, 18 May, https://www.ncregister.com/blog/public-masses-resume-in-italy-but-not-without-controversy. Accessed 23 April 2023.

Perrin, J. and Vasco Rocca, S. (1999), *s.v. gants pontificaux*, Paris: Éd. du Patrimoine, p. 330.

Pickstock, C. (1998), *After Writing: On Liturgical Consummation of Philosophy*, Oxford: Blackwell Publishers.

Roszak, P. (2020), 'Mute sacrum: Faiths and its relation to heritage on the Camino de Santiago', *Religions*, 11:2, art. 70.

Scott, H. R. (2020), 'Worship in a post-lockdown context: A ritual-liturgical perspective', *HTS Teologiese Studies/Theological Studies*, 76:1, p. a6112, https://doi.org/10.4102/hts.v76i1.6112.

Tytarenko, V. and Bogachevska, I. (2021), 'Religious "Covid fundamentalism" in Eastern and Central Europe: Challenges and lessons', *Occasional Papers on Religion in Eastern Europe*, 41:1, art. 4.

Welte, B. (1952), *Vom Wesen und Unwesen der Religion*, Frankfurt am Main: Knecht.

4

Protesting in Defence of Human Rights in the Time of Pandemic: Freedom of Assembly and COVID-19

Grażyna Baranowska and Aleksandra Gliszczyńska-Grabias

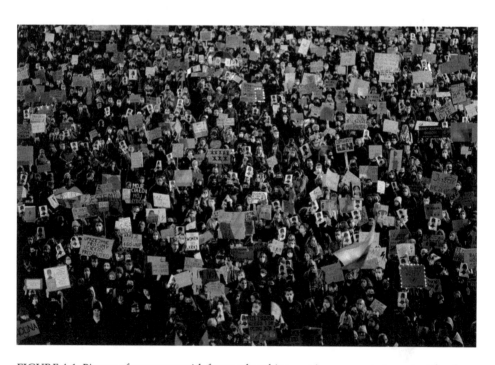

FIGURE 4.1: Picture of protesters with facemasks taking part in mass protests against the abortion judgement in Poland in October 2020, Łukasz Cynalewski, Gazeta Wyborcza.

Introduction

The closing scene of Camus' novel *The Plague* describes the cheering crowd that celebrates the end of the pandemic:

> And, indeed, as he listened to the cries of joy rising from the town, Rieux remembered that such joy is always imperilled. He knew what those jubilant crowds did not know but could have learned from books: that the plague bacillus never dies or disappears for good; that it can lie dormant for years and years in furniture and linen-chests, that it bides its time in bedrooms, cellars, trunks, and bookshelves; and that perhaps the day would come when, for the bane and enlightening of men, it roused up its rats again and sent them forth to die in a happy city.
> (Camus 2017: 297)

The gathering of all the citizens of the city of Oran, coming together again after a long time of enforced isolation, is symbolic: it is one of the most visible proofs of going back to 'normal life', going back to societal behaviours, going back to being together. And even though the metaphorical warning of the plague coming back keeps the reader away from the comfort of closing the book and putting it back on the shelf, the moment of the survivors' reunion is, at the same time, a moment of hope and relief. Perhaps, as Camus tells us, just a very brief one.

As the history of 'the plagues' teaches us, during pandemics, taking part in gatherings should be avoided. We are urged – or ordered – to stay home and refrain even from meeting anyone else except our household members. It causes stress, frustration and discomfort, but is generally accepted as one of the methods of limiting the social interactions that are responsible for further infections. However, from the beginning of the COVID-19 pandemic, all over the world, huge, unprecedented in-person protests took place. These include the protests in the United States after the murder of George Floyd in May 2020 (Taylor 2021), in Belarus after the blatant electoral manipulation in August 2020 (HRW 2021) and in the Indian farmers' protest of 2020–21, in which millions of citizens participated (Mashal et al. 2021). In Poland, we took part and are still taking part in numerous protests, including those in support of the harassed judges and the independence of the judiciary, those to defend women and their reproductive rights, those against homophobia and transphobia and so on. In fact, we have probably never attended as many protests as we did in 2020/21. While fearing for the life and health of ourselves and our families, we regularly – during some weeks, daily – put on our facemasks and marched in protests with others.

It is paradoxical that so many protests took place during a pandemic, particularly since assemblies were seriously limited and, in many places, completely forbidden. In March 2020, the World Health Organization declared a state of pandemic, and Poland, the country in which both authors were living during that moment, instituted a lockdown. The Polish government, just like other governments, introduced many restrictions that aimed to limit the spread of COVID-19. Some of the restrictions were quite unusual, such as the prohibition against entering forests, with exceptions being granted only to hunters. Others were more common, such as the obligation to wear facemasks or a ban on public gatherings. However, the prohibition on gatherings and public protests was later found to be introduced without a proper legal basis (see Section 5 of this chapter).

What makes people, individuals and large crowds take part in protests during a pandemic? Why would they be willing to expose themselves to a virus and violate a prohibition in order to protest? In the following parts of this chapter, we will try to answer these questions by explaining why we, among millions of other Poles, chose to protest and what our motivations were. We begin this chapter with a general introduction to freedom of assembly guarantees that are enshrined in the Polish Constitution and in international human rights law, arguing that a complete prohibition on protests during a pandemic cannot be justified. Next, we move on to the description of the human rights violations and the assault on the rule of law and independent judiciary by the Polish authorities that caused the reaction of the society in the form of massive protests. The fourth section points out the reaction of the state towards the protesters and the unlawful measures used to suppress civil society's mobilization, with the abuse of legal tools implemented in the context of COVID-19 prevention. Here, we concentrate mostly on the actions taken by the police that, in many cases, should be described as nothing but a pure, illegal abuse of power. The fifth section turns to the positive and encouraging aspects of the events, including the legal fight against human rights violations caused by the actions undertaken against the protesters. The mobilization of legal aid and representation of victims in front of the courts, as well as the challenges of certain laws imposed by the state in the context of the right to assembly in the time of the pandemic, were of unprecedented scope and success. The chapter ends with conclusions.

The right to assembly and its limitations

The right to assembly constitutes a fundamental freedom that is strictly connected to the very essence of democracy. It is closely linked to freedom of speech and freedom of association. It is also with this particular freedom that limitations can take the form of the most drastic and memorable events, such as the 1989 brutal pacification of the Tiananmen Square protests in China (Lim 2014) or the communist crimes committed against Polish miners during the 'Wujek' coal mine protests in 1981 (Nowara 2011).

The Polish Constitution guarantees the right to assembly in Article 57, which stipulates that 'The freedom of peaceful assembly and participation in such assemblies shall be ensured to everyone. Limitations upon such freedoms may be imposed by statute' (Constitution of the Republic of Poland 1997). Its particular aspects have often been tackled by the Polish courts, including by the Polish Constitutional Tribunal (CT); for example, in September 2014, the CT issued a landmark judgement regarding the freedom to organize peaceful assemblies (*Wyrok Trybunału Konstytucyjnego* 2014). The Tribunal questioned, inter alia, the lack of regulations on the so-called spontaneous assemblies, defects of the appeal procedure against the ban on holding an assembly and the principle of 'separating' assemblies held at the same time in the vicinity of the principal assembly. This positive attitude, which actually widened and strengthened the protections of those who wished to gather together, was later challenged by the decisions of the Polish government.

The right to assembly is recognized in all major human rights treaties. At the UN level, the International Covenant on Civil and Political Rights Article 21 obliges states to recognize and guarantee the right to assembly. The exercise of this right can be restricted in conformity with the law and only when necessary in a democratic society for strictly listed reasons, including the protection of public health. Under specific circumstances, states can derogate from the right to assembly; however, according to the Human Rights Committee, states should only do this if they can attain their objectives by imposing restrictions in conformity with the conditions set forth in Article 21 (UN Human Rights Committee 2020). The UN has also addressed the specific issue of limiting rights and freedoms specifically *vis-à-vis* the COVID-19 pandemic addressed (UN 2020).

In the statement of UN human rights experts, including mandate holders of the special procedures, it has been stressed that

> [w]hile we recognize the severity of the current health crisis and acknowledge that the use of emergency powers is allowed by international law in response to significant threats, we urgently remind States that any emergency responses to the coronavirus must be proportionate, necessary and non-discriminatory.

One of the most important paragraphs of their statement, which is also most relevant to the present chapter, stresses that emergency conduct introduced to fight the COVID-19 outbreak should not be used as a basis to target particular groups, minorities, or individuals. It should not function as a cover for repressive action under the guise of protecting health nor should it be used to silence the work of human rights defenders.

This clearly relates to the situation we have witnessed in Poland, where selected groups and selected issues within the human rights agenda have been intentionally and excessively used by the authorities to silence the protesters.

The EU Charter of Fundamental Rights sets guarantees for freedom of assembly in its Art. 12, Para. 1, which reads,

> Everyone has the right to freedom of peaceful assembly and to freedom of association at all levels, in particular in political, trade union and civic matters, which implies the right of everyone to form and to join trade unions for the protection of his or her interests.
>
> (EU 2000)

Moreover, within the human rights protection system of the Council of Europe, the right to assembly has been addressed many times by the European Court of Human Rights (ECtHR), also in the context of its possible limitations. For example, in one of the latest cases decided by the ECtHR in regard to freedom of assembly, its violation has been found in the case of two applicants who argued that their participation in a rally had been peaceful and that the use of force against them had therefore been unlawful and unjustified (*Zakharov and Varzhabetyan v. Russia* 2006). In another case, the ECtHR decided that Article 11 of the European Convention of Human Rights and Fundamental Freedoms had been breached as the result of a ban ordered by the police. The police banned the applicant, who organized a demonstration in Istanbul to protest against plans for a certain type of prison, from reading a press statement at the end of the demonstration (*Oya Ataman v. Turkey* 2006). Some of the core elements of the Strasbourg Court's understanding of this freedom are to be found in its judgement in *Lashmankin and Others v. Russia* (2017), where the ECtHR addressed various aspects of time, place and manner restrictions of political protests in Russia, organized and conducted in order to manifest citizens' objections to the various human rights violations conducted by the Russian authorities, including in the context of fraudulent elections.

Some of the cases concerning specific limitations on the freedom of assembly on the ground of the COVID-19 pandemic have already been communicated to the relevant governments. In the case initiated against Croatia, the applicants argue that the restrictions and prohibitions introduced by the authorities in relation to the COVID-19 pandemic (namely, the decisions prohibiting leaving places of domicile and residence, save in exceptional circumstances and with authorization, prohibiting public gatherings comprising more than five people and suspending religious gatherings), violated freedom of assembly, among other alleged human rights and freedoms violations (*Magdić v. Croatia* 2021). Another communicated case was initiated by the applicant, who, as a result of the introduced bans, was not able to hold an assembly that was already planned and organized (Communauté genevoise d'action syndicale [CGAS] v. Switzerland 2020). There was also no other possibility for the applicants to participate directly in the public sphere. The decision of the ECtHR in these cases is awaited with impatience, as it will set forth the judicial line that is crucial for the interpretation of the European human rights standard on the freedom of assembly.

Another aspect worth noting here is the phenomenon of civil disobedience. In their joint guidelines on freedom of assembly, the Venice Commission and the Office for Democratic Institutions and Human Rights (ODIHR) of the OSCE addressed this issue as follows:

> There are times when the manner in which an assembly is conducted intentionally violates the law in a fashion that organizers and/or participants believe will amplify or otherwise assist in the communication of their message. This is commonly referred to as 'civil disobedience'. Those who engage in civil disobedience often strive to do so in a peaceful manner and commonly accept the duly prescribed legal penalty. State responses, including arrests and penalties, should be proportional to the respective offences.
>
> (Venice Commission and OSCE ODIHR 2020: 7)

Thus, even assuming that the limitations and bans introduced by Polish authorities were lawful, the reaction of Polish civil society should be seen as a manifestation of civil disobedience in its most noble form.

Protesting in Poland during the COVID-19 pandemic in defence of human rights

When the COVID-19 pandemic hit, the checks and balances characteristic of the separation of powers in a democratic state had already been dismantled in Poland for some time. Wojciech Sadurski famously framed the process as a 'constitutional breakdown' (Sadurski 2019). One of the characteristics of the disregard for the rule of law was adopting laws overnight and adopting executive orders instead of laws of Parliaments. Another is the attempt to take over the judiciary. All of these trends are exemplified in the situations that played out in the protests we took part in during COVID-19.

One of the very first moves of the new government in 2015 was not the non-appointment of the judges elected to the CT, but instead appointing new judges in violation of the law (so-called 'doubles'). Shortly after that, one of the new persons elected to the court, Julia Przyłębska, was appointed to be the court's president.

As stated by the European Court of Human Rights, the inclusion in the adjudicating panels of persons who have been appointed to the CT with irregularities, results in the CT not being a 'tribunal established by law' (Xero Flor w Polsce sp. z o.o. v. Poland 2021).

In October 2020, a decision of the CT under Julia Przyłębska led to the largest protests since 1990, commonly called the *Women's Strike*. The decision severely restricted very harsh abortion regulations by making it impossible to abort malformed fetuses (see Gliszczyńska-Grabias and Sadurski 2021; Wyrzykowski 2020; Soniewicka 2021; Sękowska-Kozłowska 2021; Grzebyk 2021). Protests began right after the ruling and continued for several weeks in most Polish towns and cities – despite the prohibition. We (the authors) also participated in the 'walks', as they were called: walks, unlike gatherings, were allowed. We took part because we believe in women and reproductive rights, but also because the way the decision was taken exemplifies the disregard for the rule of law in Poland. Not all of the members of the CT under Julia Przyłębska who took part in the proceedings can be regarded as lawfully appointed judges of the Constitution Tribunal: three out of the thirteen persons sitting on the panel and signing off the decision had joined the Tribunal as a result of faulty elections to seats already occupied by other, properly elected judges (Szwed 2022). Furthermore, the proceedings were started by a number of MPs from the ruling party, who, instead of proposing an amendment to the law in Parliament, chose to petition the no-longer-independent court.

The mass protests were consistently broken up by the police. Messages informing the protesters that the assemblies were illegal were broadcasted through loudspeakers, cordons were placed along the route's marches, streets were blocked and tickets were issued. All of this was done based on the executive order. Legal scholars have urged from the very beginning that such a ban would need to be adopted as a law by Parliament and not issued as an executive order. This was confirmed in a July 2021 Supreme Court ruling, which concerned two participants in the so-called Women's Strike protests. The court decided that the executive motion was introduced without a proper legal basis and contrary to the Constitution (Wyrok Sądu Najwyższego w Warszawie w sprawie M. J. i S.S 2021). Thus, both the reason for the protests (a decision by the unlawfully appointed judicial body) and the way the government chose to suppress freedom of assembly (via an improperly introduced executive motion) are deeply rooted in the decline of the rule of law in Poland.

The second reason why we protested regularly during COVID-19 lies at the heart of the decline: the independence of judges. The times of the pandemic in Poland were simultaneously the times of increased attacks on the independent judiciary. The unlawful decisions of a disciplinary body within the Supreme Court of Poland, the so-called Disciplinary Chamber, taken against judges such as Paweł

Juszczyszyn or Igor Tuleya, sparked an enormous reaction that could not be fully translated into street protests, precisely because of the limitations imposed. Civil society representatives, citizens and members of judges' associations gathered in front of the building of the Supreme Court in Warsaw every time the illegal Chamber acted against the judges; however, the limitations imposed made it impossible to organize huge protests. It is interesting to note that, although other Polish courts were not proceeding because of COVID-19, the illegal Chamber was acting 'fullstream', most likely because of the lack of a full audience during their law-violating 'hearings'. This kind of lawlessness is much easier to implement without the direct, in-room presence of free media, civil society representatives and the audience: the seemingly comforting feeling that 'not many are watching' did not, however, work in the case of the Court of Justice of the European Union: the Luxemburg Court had been following these events and concluded its observations in its subsequent judgements (Pech and Kochenov 2021).

Measures taken against the protesters during the COVID-19 pandemic

During the mass protests, the police recorded massive numbers of identities of people participating and detained many of them. According to information revealed by one of the organizations legally supporting the protesters, within the first 100 days after the abortion decision of 'the CT under Julia Przyłębska', 150 people were detained for taking part in protests. In 81 cases, those people spent a night in detention, often in a city other than where the protest took place (Szpila 2021). A widespread practice during the protests was where the police would surround the protesters from all sides, only allowing those who would show their identity cards to the police to leave the space. Such a practice, for example, led to the collection of names of over 900 people during one protest held on 28 November 2020 (Karwowska 2020).

The protests were also met with disproportionate use of police force, as evidenced by reports issued by NGOs and the National Preventive Mechanism. Police brutality has been noted, both regarding persons taking part in the protests and detained persons. Police officers were reported to have used extensive force, placing protesters in handcuffs and referring to detainees in homophobic or transphobic ways. Personal checks were also reported to have been exercised in ways that violated the dignity of the detained, and the detainees reportedly had hampered access to lawyers. These developments were evident during protests that took place as early as August 2020 (triggered by the homophobic hate speech of state officials) and highlighted by the National Preventive Mechanism Report (Krajowy Mechanizm Prewencji Tortur 2020).

The police have not yet been responsive to these findings, and the situation in the autumn, following the abortion decision by the CT under Julia Przyłębska mirrored the drastic situation in the summer (Helsińska Fundacja Praw Człowieka 2021).

The detention of peaceful protesters also needs to be assessed in light of the COVID-19 pandemic. Viruses are likely to spread in closed facilities, such as places of detention. Although detaining peaceful protesters should always be a measure of last resort, during a pandemic, the likelihood of infection and transferring of the virus needs to be considered as well. In the above-described situation, this thread was clearly not considered. Overall, this may serve as an example of an anti-democratic government limiting the rights and freedoms of its opponents.

Legal response of human rights defenders

Faced with the wave of illegal actions by the police and other state organs against the protesters, Polish lawyers decided to act. They organized themselves in 'urgent reaction' groups that intervened in every case signalled to them, accompanying detainees to the police stations. This immediate pro bono legal assistance was of great importance in particular for the young people who were confronted with a system of oppression for the very first time and, in many cases, police brutality. The attitude of many Polish lawyers who decided to support the oppressed protesters was best summarized by one of them:

> My attitude could not be different towards the ongoing protests of women caused by the decision about the alleged incompatibility of some abortion regulations with the Polish Constitution (called by the ruling party and their supporters – the judgement of the Constitutional Tribunal). As a lawyer and as a citizen of the Republic of Poland, I am opposed to Thursday's decision as to its substance and procedure, or more precisely to the 'authority' by which it was taken. The adjudicating panel consisted of persons who had been appointed contrary to the law, closely related to the ruling party and who could not be attributed the quality of law and order, justice, and independence.
>
> (Gajda 2021: n.pag.)

Eventually, a very large number of individual cases were referred to the Polish courts, which generally stood firm behind constitutional rights and freedoms and international human rights guarantees. During the total ban on assemblies, the Court of Appeal in Warsaw stated:

The above legal situation raises serious doubts from the point of view of the constitutional right of citizens to assembly resulting from Art. 57 of the Polish Constitution, particularly in the context of constitutionally permissible limitations of subjective rights and the principle of proportionality contained in Art. 31 Sec. 3 of the Polish Constitution.

(*Postanowienie Sądu Apelacyjnego w Warszawie w sprawie M. J.* 2020)

The courts also noted that even if it were possible to restrict the freedom of assembly by power and on the basis of the government's ordinance, such measures could not have had the effect of prohibiting participation in assemblies, as they concerned the organization of such events (*Orzeczenie Sądu Rejonowego dla Warszawy-Śródmieścia* 2020). The police also reacted excessively in cases where smaller protests and happenings were organized, during which distance was kept and all other safety rules were complied with. As the District Court for Warszawa-Śródmieście in Warsaw pointed out:

> The accused have kept all the necessary and legally required safety measures aimed at ensuring the health safety of themselves and others and, in the Court's opinion, it cannot be claimed that this type of their behaviour could violate public order or order and justify their punishment.

However, the most significant judicial *dictum* came from the Supreme Court in July 2021, case no. IV KK 238/21 (Wyrok Sądu Najwyższego o niedopuszczalności ukarania na podstawie art 54 k.w. w związku z ograniczeniami w czasie epidemii COVID, KK 238/21 2021). It concerned the case of a demonstration in front of the local office of the Law and Justice party that took place as a reaction towards the judgement of the CT under Julia Przyłębska on abortion law. The judgement was issued as a result of a cassation appeal brought by the Polish Ombudsman, Adam Bodnar, who, from the very beginning of the COVID-19 pandemic, indicated that the government's ban on assembly during a pandemic, which was introduced by subsequent regulations, violated the essence of the constitutional freedom of assembly. As the Ombudsman argued, this actually and fully prevented citizens from effectively exercising this freedom. The Supreme Court ruled that the government introduced the ban on public gatherings without a proper legal basis – by the way of an ordinary regulation and contrary to Art. 57 and Art. 31 Sec. 3 of the Polish Constitution.

Moreover, Polish courts have also recognized cases where bans on different kinds of public gatherings were implemented in the violation of law. When, in January 2021, the number of COVID-19 infections in Poland began to increase rapidly, the government adopted a regulation that ordered the closure of discos and nightclubs

(Rada Ministrów 2020). An entrepreneur breaking this ban, who opened his disco, was fined after the sanitary inspection. In September 2021, the Provincial Court of Appeal in Gorzów Wielkopolski overturned the decisions issued in this case and discontinued the administrative proceedings, stating that the government's ordinance had been issued in violation of the law (Wyrok Wojewódzkiego Sądu Administracyjnego w Gorzowie Wielkopolskim o konstytucyjności zakazu prowadzenia dyskotek i klubów nocnych w związku z epidemią COViD-19 2021). The court indicated that pursuant to Art. 46a and Art. 46b Point 2 of the ordinance, the government was authorized to introduce 'a temporary limitation of certain scopes of business activity'. However, this authorization does not allow for the adoption of a limitation of business activity that equals prohibiting it. The restriction cannot amount to a complete prohibition. Thus, the ban on running discos and nightclubs was introduced beyond the limits of statutory authorization. The court emphasized that the legislator may interfere with the constitutional freedom of economic activity but must act using the means provided for by the Constitution itself.

All the examples outlined above prove the crucially important and essential role of judicial independence. Without it, all the efforts and engagement of the lawyers in defending the protesters and other citizens from the unlawful actions of the state would remain meaningless.

Conclusions

Unusual, turbulent times and events always demand unusual measures to counteract the dramatic consequences of the sudden turmoil. In the case of the COVID-19 pandemic, the response had to also encompass a variety of measures that strictly limited particular rights and freedoms of individuals and groups. Under such circumstances, a dilemma very often arises: Should we stand firm by the human rights protection standards or should we agree to their severe limitations? This dilemma is further deepened by a phenomenon that characterizes almost all political forces and governments: an attempt to increase their control over societies. Thus, it is often not clear whether the imposed limitations are indeed absolutely necessary measures or whether they have been introduced to consolidate power and silence the critics of those in power at a given time and place.

Such is the case of freedom of assembly and protest limitations implemented in Poland during the COVID-19 pandemic in order to stop the protests held by the LGBTQ+ community and the massive protests against the unlawful decision of the illegally acting CT under Julia Przyłębska in the so-called abortion case. The courts' interpretations of the decisions and orders imposed against the protesters, including their detention, have exposed the unlawful, unconstitutional character of the introduced measures. What is more, the decisions and orders seem to stand in violation of the binding international human rights law provisions that were not 'suspended' during the pandemic.

The case of Poland clearly indicates the risks that are at stake when it comes to anti-democratic governments being given tools to limit the rights and freedoms of their opponents, with a justification that is difficult to reject in a time of social fear and uncertainty. At the same time, the events outlined in this chapter prove that pro-democratic societies are ready to stand in defence of human rights despite all limitations, difficulties and personal risks. It is thanks to such an attitude that the world has heard about the blatant violation of women's rights, the acts of violence against the LGBTQ+ community and the attempts to complete the process of destroying the independent Polish judiciary. All actions taken by civil society in this context should be perceived as a symbol of the fight for human rights and for the continued belonging of Poland to the universal and European systems of human rights protection.

REFERENCES

Camus, Albert (2017), *The Plague*, London: Penguin.

Communauté genevoise d'action syndicale (CGAS) v. Switzerland (2020), application no. 21881/20.

Constitution of the Republic of Poland (1997), 'Chapter II: The freedoms, rights and obligations of persons and citizens', https://www.senat.gov.pl/en/about-the-senate/konstytucja/chapter-ii/. Accessed 27 March 2023.

EU (2000), 'Charter of fundamental rights of the European Union', *Official Journal of the European Union*, C 326/391, https://www.europarl.europa.eu/charter/pdf/text_en.pdf. Accessed 27 March 2020.

Gajda, Michał (2021), 'Wspieramy Strajk Kobiet', https://gajda-adwokat.pl/wspieramy-strajk-kobiet/. Accessed 27 March 2023.

Gliszczyńska-Grabias, Aleksandra and Sadurski, Wojciech (2021), 'The judgment that wasn't (BUT WHICH NEARLY BROUGHT Poland to a Standstill): "Judgment' of the Polish Constitutional Tribunal of 22 October 2020, K1/20, 2021"', *European Constitutional Law Review*, 17:1, pp. 130–53.

Grzebyk, Piotr (2021), 'Ogólnopolski Strajk Kobiet, aborcja i prawo do strajku', *Państwo i Prawo*, 906:8, pp. 184–95.

Helsińska Fundacja Praw Człowieka (2021), 'Impact of the coronavirus pandemic on the criminal justice system. Freedom of assembly – update', February, https://hfhr.pl/upload/2022/01/freedom-of-assembly-brief_.pdf. Accessed 27 March 2023.

HRW (2021), 'Belarus: Unprecedented crackdown. Arrests, torture of peaceful protesters follow disputed election', *Human Rights Watch*, 13 January, https://www.hrw.org/news/2021/01/13/belarus-unprecedented-crackdown. Accessed 27 March 2023.

Karwowska, Anita (2020), 'Strajk Kobiet i prof. Płatek radzą obywatelom. Co zrobić, gdy policja ogranicza nasze prawa', *Gazeta Wyborcza*, 2 December, https://wyborcza.pl/7,162657,26566398,strajk-kobiet-radzi-obywatelom-co-zrobic-gdy-policja-ogranicza.html. Accessed 27 March 2023.

Krajowy Mechanizm Prewencji Tortur (2020), *Raport z wizytacji 'ad hoc' pomieszczeń dla osób zatrzymanych lub doprowadzonych do wytrzeźwienia, znajdujących się w jednostkach podległych Komendzie Stołecznej Policji*, KMP.570.5.2020.MK, Warszawa, http://surl.li/fvwsq. Accessed 27 March 2023.

Lashmankin and Others v. Russia (2017), Application nos. 57818/09 and 14 others.

Lim, Louisa (2014), *The People's Republic of Amnesia: Tiananmen Revisited*, Oxford: Oxford University Press.

Magdić v. Croatia (2021), Application no. 17578/20.

Mashal, Mujib, Schmall, Emily and Goldman, Russell (2021), 'Why are farmers protesting in India?' *The New York Times*, 21 January, https://www.nytimes.com/2021/01/27/world/asia/india-farmer-protest.html. Accessed 27 March 2023.

Ministrów, Rada (2020), *Rozrpozsądzienie. w sprawie ustanowienia określonych ograniczeń, nakazawa i zakazów w związku z wystąpieniem stanu epidemii* ('Regulation of the Council of Ministers as of 21 December 2020 on the establishment of certain restrictions, orders and prohibitions in connection with an epidemic'), 21 December, Dz.U. 2020 poz. 2316, https://isap.sejm.gov.pl/isap.nsf/DocDetails.xsp?id=WDU20200002316. Accessed 27 March 2023.

Nowara, Tomasz (2011), Kopalnia 'Wujek' 13–16 grudnia 1981 r. W hołdzie tym, którzy odeszli … za wcześnie ('Mine "Wujek" December 13–16, 1981 In tribute to those who left … too soon'), Społeczny Komitet Pamięci Górników KWK 'Wujek' Poległych 16 Grudnia 1981 r., Katowice.

Orzeczenie Sądu Rejonowego dla Warszawy-Śródmieścia (2020), V W 1083/20.

Oya Ataman v. Turkey (2006), Application no. 74552/01.

Pech, Laurent and Kochenov, Dimitry (2021), 'Respect for the rule of law in the case law of the European Court of Justice: A casebook overview of key judgements since the Portuguese judges case', *SIEPS*, Stockholm, https://www.sieps.se/en/publications/2021/respect-for-the-rule-of-law-in-the-case-law-of-the-european-court-of-justice/. Accessed 28 March 2023.

Postanowienie Sądu Apelacyjnego w Warszawie w sprawie M. J. (2020), VI Acz 339/20.

Sadurski, Wojciech (2019), *Poland's Constitutional Breakdown*, Oxford: Oxford University Press.

Sękowska-Kozłowska, Katarzyna (2021), 'Dopuszczalność przerywania ciąży ze względów embriopatologicznych w świetle Konwencji ONZ o prawach osób niepełnosprawnych i praktyki Komitetu ONZ do spraw praw osób niepełnosprawnych', *Państwo i Prawo*, 906:8, pp. 167–83.

Soniewicka, Monika (2021), 'Spór o dopuszczalność przerywania ciąży z perspektywy etycznej i filozoficznoprawnej (komentarz do wyroku TK w sprawie K 1/20)', *Państwo i Prawo*, 906:8, pp. 6–23.

Szpila (2021), 'Raport (anty)represyjny – 100 dni protestu', Facebook, 21 February, https://www.facebook.com/kolektywszpila/posts/136721888271686. Accessed 27 March 2023.

Szwed, Marcin (2022), 'The Polish constitutional tribunal crisis from the perspective of the European Convention on Human Rights: EctHR 7 May 2021, No. 4907/18, Xero Flor w Polsce sp. Z o.o. v Poland', *European Constitutional Law Review*, 18:1, pp. 132–54.

Taylor, Derrick Bryson (2021), 'George Floyd protests: A timeline', *The New York Times*, 2 October, https://www.nytimes.com/article/george-floyd-protests-timeline.html. Accessed 27 March 2023.

UN (2020), 'COVID-19: States should not abuse emergency measures to suppress human rights UN experts', *United Nations*, 16 March, https://www.ohchr.org/EN/NewsEvents/Pages/DisplayNews.aspx?NewsID=25722&LangID=E. Accessed 27 March 2020.

UN Human Rights Committee (2020), *General Comment No. 37 on the Right of Peaceful Assembly (Article 21)*, CCPR/C/GC/37, 17 September, https://www.ohchr.org/en/documents/general-comments-and-recommendations/general-comment-no-37-article-21-right-peaceful. Accessed 27 March 2023.

Venice Commission and the OSCE ODIHR (2020), *Guidelines on Freedom of Peaceful Assembly*, tCDL-AD (2019)017rev, p. 7.

Wyrok Sądu Najwyższego o niedopuszczalności ukarania na podstawie art. 54 k.w. w związku z ograniczeniami w czasie epidemii COVID (2021), KK 238/21, http://www.sn.pl/sites/orzecznictwo/orzeczenia3/iv%20kk%20238-21.pdf. Accessed 27 March 2023.

Wyrok Sądu Najwyższego w Warszawie w sprawie M. J. i S.S (2021), IV KK 238/21, http://www.sn.pl/sites/orzecznictwo/orzeczenia3/iv%20kk%20238-21.pdf. Accessed 28 March 2023.

Wyrok Trybunału Konstytucyjnego (2014), K 44/12, https://isap.sejm.gov.pl/isap.nsf/download.xsp/WDU20140001327/T/D20141327TK.pdf. Accessed 27 March 2023.

Wyrok Wojewódzkiego Sądu Administracyjnego w Gorzowie Wielkopolskim o konstytucyjności zakazu prowadzenia dyskotek i klubów nocnych w związku z epidemią COVID-19 (2021), II SA/Go 564/21.

Wyrzykowski, Mirosław (2020), 'Waking up demons: Bad legislation for an even worse case', *European Papers*, 5:3, pp. 1171–89.

Xero Flor w Polsce sp. z o.o. v. Poland (2021), Application no. 4907/18.

Zakharov and Varzhabetyan v. Russia (2006), Applications nos. 35880/14 and 75926/17.

PLAGUE IN HISTORY

5

Recounting the Plague in Sixteenth and Seventeenth-Century London

Charles Giry-Deloison

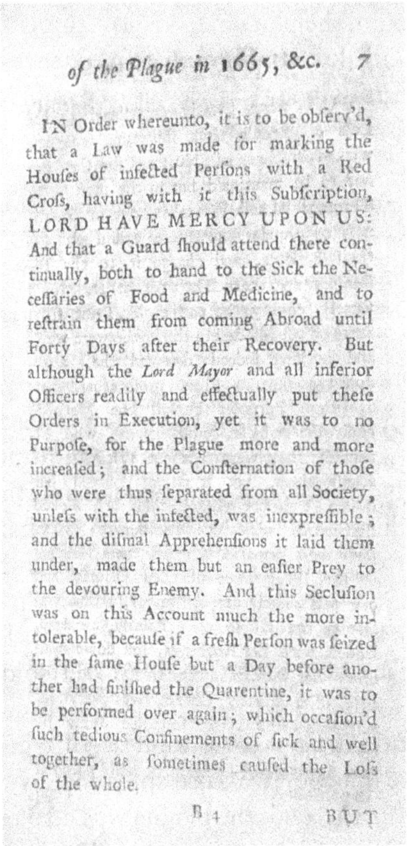
of the Plague in 1665, &c. 7

IN Order whereunto, it is to be obſerv'd, that a Law was made for marking the Houſes of infected Perſons with a Red Croſs, having with it this Subſcription, LORD HAVE MERCY UPON US: And that a Guard ſhould attend there continually, both to hand to the Sick the Neceſſaries of Food and Medicine, and to reſtrain them from coming Abroad until Forty Days after their Recovery. But although the *Lord Mayor* and all inferior Officers readily and effectually put theſe Orders in Execution, yet it was to no Purpoſe, for the Plague more and more increaſed; and the Conſternation of thoſe who were thus ſeparated from all Society, unleſs with the infected, was inexpreſſible; and the diſmal Apprehenſions it laid them under, made them but an eaſier Prey to the devouring Enemy. And this Seclusion was on this Account much the more intolerable, becauſe if a freſh Perſon was ſeized in the ſame Houſe but a Day before another had finiſhed the Quarentine, it was to be performed over again; which occaſion'd ſuch tedious Confinements of ſick and well together, as ſometimes cauſed the Loſs of the whole.

B 4 BUT

FIGURE 5.1: Nathaniel HODGES, *Loimologia: or, an Historical Account of the Plague in London in 1665* [...], London, printed for E. Bell and J. Osborn, 1721, 3rd ed., p. 7. Paris: Bibliothèque nationale de France, 8-TD53-190.

Plague was a regular fixture of life in sixteenth and seventeenth-century England – like it was in many parts of the world – and no city was immune from it, London least of all. It seems that in England, plague was not endemic but imported from the continent in the wake of each wave of infection that spread through Europe. Nevertheless, in infected areas, plague could linger on for years, if not decades, thus meaning that it was really never absent from any part of the country between 1485 and 1665; only the years 1612–24 and 1654–64 seem to have been free of the disease. In London, for example, after a respite in 1604–05, there was a resurgence of the disease from 1606 until at least 1610 (Creighton 1891: 493–94). On several occasions, relatively short but extremely violent outbursts decimated the population, notably in London in 1563, 1578, 1593, 1603, 1625, 1636 and 1665 (Slack [1985] 1990: 145–47). The fear, the deaths, the desolation, the lack of adequate remedy and the feeling of helplessness led to a vast production of literature on and around the plague, from governmental orders, sermons and medical treatises that aimed to contain the consequences of the epidemic to *ars moriendi* and other 'crafts of dying', as well as to pamphlets and diaries recounting the plague.

The purpose of this chapter is to compare two first-hand accounts of the plague in London in the early and mid-seventeenth century, those of Thomas Dekker's *The Wonderfull Yeare* on the plague of 1603 (Dekker [1603] 1884), and Nathaniel Hodges' *Loimologia, or, An Historical Account of the Plague in London in 1665* (Hodges 1720), with the aim of understanding how two Londoners, half a century apart, described the plague using two very different literary genres: a pamphlet (*The Wonderfull Yeare*) and a medical treatise (*Loimologia*).

The plague that devastated London in 1603–04 had reached England in the early months of the previous year through the ports of Kingston upon Hull (Yorkshire) and Great Yarmouth (Norfolk) on the east coast, and those of Dartmouth and Plymouth (Devon) on the south, before spreading haphazardly along rivers and roads to most parts of the country: Chester in September 1602, Stamford in Lincolnshire in December, Oxford in July 1603, Bristol in August, etc. (Creighton 1891: 474–92, 496; Slack [1985] 1990: 66). A few years later, John Stow laid the responsibility for the resurgence of the disease on the soldiers returning from the Low Countries: 'In the former yere to wit, 1602. the plague of peft. being great in Holland, Zealand, and other the Low Countries, and many souldiers returning thence into England, the infection was also spread in divers parts of this Realme' (Stow 1631: 833). By March 1603, the plague was also reaching the outskirts of London. On the 25th the first deaths were recorded in the parish of Stepney, which lay a few miles east of the City (Creighton 1891: 473; Slack [1985] 1990: 150). This caused alarm in London: on 18 April, the lord mayor, Sir Robert Lee, wrote to the Privy Council asking what measures were to be taken 'to prevent the spread of the plague in the counties of Middlesex and Surrey' (Creighton 1891: 493). No doubt the funeral of Elizabeth I, which was to be held on the 28th, was high on the authorities' preoccupations, and the risk of plague-infested crowds entering the City to watch the procession was a seriously worrying prospect. A month later, on 29 May, an order was given to gentlemen to depart the Court and City on account of the plague (Green 1857: I, n° 98) and, on Sunday 25 July, the King's coronation route had to be changed as he could no longer pass through the City; all the pageants had to be performed between Westminster Bridge and the Abbey (Green 1857: II, 18 July; Stow 1631: 827). As in 1579, 1592 and 1593, a book of plague orders was published in July 1603. It was a reprint of the one of 1579 (and of the subsequent runs), only updated to take into account the change of monarch, and it contained two parts: the actual orders and medical prescriptions (*Advice*) drawn up by the College of Physicians (Anon. 1603; Slack [1985] 1990: 209–10).

In London, in the early sixteenth century, the causes of death started to be recorded weekly by the parish clerks and sent to the municipal authorities and to the King by the Company of Parish Clerks in order to warn of the onset of plague and other diseases. The plague orders specifically instructed that, in every parish, several persons should be appointed to:

'viewe the bodies of all such as shall die, before they be suffered to be buried, and to certifie the minister of the Church and Church-warden, or other principall officers, or their substitutes of what probable disease the sayd persons died', and that the justices of peace should be informed every week of those who are infected but did not die and those who did and of what cause, and that 'a particular booke kept by the Clerke of the Peace or some such like.

(Anon. 1603: paragraph 4 and 9)

By 1563, these 'bills of mortality' were being returned by the 96 (97 in 1603) parishes within the walls of the City and the sixteen parishes outside the walls but within, or partly within, the liberties of the City (Bridewell Precinct, St. Andrew Holborn, St. Bartholomew the Great, St. Bartholomew the Less, St. Botolph without Aldersgate, St. Botolph without Aldgate, St. Botolph without Bishopsgate, St. Bride Fleet Street, St. Dunstan in the West, St. George Southwark, St. Giles out Cripplegate, St. Olave Southwark, St. Saviour Southwark, St. Sepulchre, St. Thomas Southwark, Trinity Minories) (Creighton 1891: 662). From 1603, another group of parishes in Middlesex and Surrey, known as the 'out-parishes', also returned their bills of mortality to the City authorities; this group grew from nine (St. Clement Danes, St. Giles-in-the-Fields, St. James Clerkenwell, St. Katharine by the Tower, St. Leonard Shoreditch, St. Magdalen Bermondsey, St. Martin-in-the-Fields, St. Paul Covent Garden, Whitechapel) (Creighton 1891: 662) to sixteen in 1636, when seven 'distant parishes' were added, and to seventeen in 1647 (Hackney, Lambeth, Rotherhithe, St. Margaret's Westminster, St. Mary Islington, St. Mary Newington, St. Mary Savoy, Stepney) (Creighton 1891: 663; Slack [1985] 1990: 150, 374 n. 5).

The surviving bills of mortality and parish registers show that the chronology of the 1603 plague followed the usual pattern: the number of weekly deaths by plague slowly increased from mid May to the end of June, then accelerated throughout the summer with a peak in mid August–mid September, before decreasing from mid November onwards, though nevertheless remaining high. As always, it is very difficult to give precise numbers, as the data are incomplete and, in some instances, not particularly reliable (Slack [1985] 1990: 375, n. 15). Nevertheless, the table drawn up by Charles Creighton using the available figures from different sources shows that, in the City and Liberties parishes, three of the 108 deaths recorded on 17 March were due to the plague (2.8%), 59 of the 144 on 15 June (41%), 263 of the 445 on 7 July (59%), and in August, September and early October, plague accounted for between 78 and 91% of all deaths. In the out-parishes, for which figures are available only for 28 July–20 October, the percentages are even higher: between 80.5 and 94 (Creighton 1891: 476). To these numbers can be added the 1,375 deaths from all causes in the City and Liberties from 17 December 1602 to 10 March 1603. Unfortunately, Creighton does not give those from plague, only writing 'having been mostly non-plague deaths'. On the basis of these data, there were at least 38,567 deaths in London in 1603, the plague accounting for slightly more than 30,519 of them (79.13%). As Creighton pointed out, this can only be a low estimate, notably because there are no returns for the weeks before 28 July from the nine out-parishes. This estimation tallies with contemporary ones. In his *Annales*, John Stow writes:

> in the City of London, and liberties thereof, it [the plague] so increased, that in the space of one whole yeare, to wit, from the 23. of December 1602. unto the 22. of December, 1603. there died of al diseases (as was weekly accompted by the parish Clarks and so certified to the King) 38244. whereof of the Plague. 30578.
>
> (Stow 1631: 833)

The anonymous author *of Reflections on the Weekly Bills of Mortality, so far as they relate to all the Plagues which have happened in London from the Year 1502 to the Great Plague in 1665*, gives the following figures for March to December 1603 derived from the bills of mortality: 37,294 burials of which 30,561 were due to the plague (Anon. 1721b: 53). Nevertheless, Paul Slack, basing himself on more recent works, gives slightly different numbers: 31,861 burials in the City and Liberties, 26,350 of them being due to the plague (82.7%). Reported to an estimated total population of 141,000, the plague mortality rate was an impressive 17.8% (Slack [1985] 1990: 151).

The geographical and social distribution of deaths by plague shows that the worst affected parishes were the three big liberties ones, east and north of the City (St. Botolph without Aldgate, St. Botolph without Bishopsgate and St. Giles out Cripplegate) and those in the City which were adjacent to the walls in the north (All Hallows on the wall) and along the riverside to the east of the City (St. Dunstan in the River, St. Michael Crooked Lane, All Hallows the Less), whilst those the least affected laid in the centre of the City (Slack [1985] 1990: figure 6.4 155, based on the parish registers). The bills of mortality published in 1721 in *A Collection*[...] (Anon. 1721a: 67–68), for the year 1603, show very high mortality rates due to the plague also in the parishes of St. Peter the Poor and St. Stephen Coleman Street in the north of City under the wall and St. Peter Paul Wharf along the Thames to the west. This mirrors the distribution of the poorest and richest parishes in the City and Liberties, the poorest also by 1603 being the most populated and where the growth of population was the quickest. According to Peter Slack, 'By 1600 [...] the population in the poor parishes was probably five times that in the rich, and by 1660 it may have been eight times greater' (Slack [1985] 1990: 158–62). In other words, plague was the most virulent – not only in absolute numbers but also relatively to the central and rich parishes – in the poorest and most populated parishes where living conditions (overcrowded and poor housing), degraded environment and extreme poverty were recipes for disaster.

The plague of 1665 followed a very similar chronological and geographical pattern, with a first outbreak in Great Yarmouth in November 1664 (the port traded with the Netherlands, where plague was again rife) before it hit London's suburbs in 1665. In May 1666, Nathaniel Hodges (see *infra*) published an account of the plague in which he also considered that the 1665 visitation came from the Low Countries:

> After a most strict and serious Inquiry, by undoubted Testimonies, I find that this *Pest* was communicated to us from the *Netherlands* by way of Contagion; and if most probable Relations deceive me not, it came from and from *Smyrna* to *Holland* in a parcel of infected Goods.
> (Hodges [1666] 1721: 14–15)

Nevertheless, there were two differences with the 'visitation' of 1603: it was much more restricted spatially and the worst outbreaks in the provinces happened in 1666, after that in London (Slack [1985] 1990: table 3.4 63, 68–69; Creighton 1891: 680–91). On a more local level, another difference from 1603 is that the first London parishes infected lay at the west and north-west of the City, and all contemporary accounts mention the progression of the epidemic through the City from west to east, which is corroborated by the available data. Thus, William Boghurst, an apothecary in the parish of St. Giles-in-the-Fields, noted:

> The plague fell first upon the highest ground, for our parish [St. Giles-in-the-Fields] is the highest ground about London, and the best air, and was first infected. Highgate, Hampstead and Acton also all shared in it. From the west end of the town it gradually insinuated and crept down Holborn and the Strand, and then into the City, and at last to the east end of the suburbs, so that it was half a year at the west end of the city [...] before the east end and Stepney was infected, which was about the middle of July.
>
> (Creighton 1891: 656)

Sixty years later, in his fact-based fictional account of the plague in London (*Journal of the Plague Year [...] in 1665*), Daniel Defoe (1722) wrote:

> It was now mid-July, and the plague which had chiefly raged at the other end of the town, and as I said before, in the parishes of St Giles's, St Andrew's, Holbourn, and towards Westminster, began now to come eastward towards the part where I lived. It was to be observed, indeed, that it did not come straight on toward us; for the City, that is to say within the walls, was indifferent healthy still [...] It was very strange to observe that in this particular week, from the 4th to the 13th July, when, as I have observed, there died near 400 of the plague in the two parishes of St Martin's and St Giles' in the Fields only, there died in the parish of Aldgate but four, in the parish of Whitechapel three, and in the parish of Stepney but one.
>
> (Creighton 1891: 657)

In the City and Liberties, the parishes most affected were practically the same as those in 1603, as were those the least affected. According to the table constructed by Charles Creighton from the bills of mortality for all of London, the number of deaths by plague slowly increased from the end of May until the end of June and then rose sharply, peaking from the end of August to the end of September (a month later than in 1603) before, very slowly, decreasing. As in 1603, numbers remained high in December, with a little surge at the end of the month. Similarly, not only were the numbers of deaths very high, but also, during the peak, they represented over 80% of all deaths and still over 50% at the end of the year. Though the number of deaths by plague was much higher in the very populated suburbs than in the 97 parishes of the City, they represented a very similar percentage of all deaths (70% in the suburbs, 65% in the City). All in all, according to

Creighton, there were 97,306 deaths in the whole of London, 68,596 due to the plague (70.5%) (Creighton 1891: 662). Paul Slack has slightly different figures: 80,696 deaths in all, 55,797 by plague, but the percentage is nearly identical (69%). Based on Slack's figures and reported to the estimated population of 459,000 inhabitants (City, liberties and out-parishes), the plague mortality rate was 12.15% (Slack [1985] 1990: 151). The comparison with the 'visitation' of 1603 is difficult due to the difference in the area covered by the mortality bills (much bigger in 1665) and to the incomplete data for some parishes, but what is clearly apparent is that the plague of 1665 killed more Londoners (which owned it the name of 'Great Plague') but, proportionally, less of London's population than in 1603.

Thomas Dekker (c.1572–1632) was born in London, probably in 1570, but nothing is known of his early life. The first mention of his name as an author appears in the *Diary* of the theatrical manager Philip Henslowe for January 1598, by which time Dekker was imprisoned in the Poultry Compter (London). He was sent to prison again in late 1598 or early 1599, Henslowe paying for his release on both occasions. A further brush with the law came in 1613 when he was sent to the King's Bench prison until 1616, probably for debt. Dekker was a very prolific writer of pamphlets, plays and poetry, which met with some success, many of his works running into several editions, some well after his death (Stephen and Lee 1885–1900, vol. 14). On several occasions, he collaborated with other playwrights, such as John Day (1574–c.1638), Ben Jonson (1572–1637) – with whom he quickly fell out and quarreled– John Marston (c.1575–1634) or Philip Massinger (1583–1640). Dekker turned to pamphleteering in 1603, when the theatres were closed due to the plague. Most of his pamphlets deal with life in Jacobean London, particularly of its underworld, and he took a particular interest in the ravages of the plague in the City, writing six known so-called plague pamphlets: *The Wonderfull Yeare* (1603), *News from Graves-end* (Dekker 1604a), *The Meeting of Gallants* (1604, maybe in collaboration with or by Thomas Middleton; Dekker 1604b), *The Seven Deadly Sins* (Dekker 1606) and three on the plague of 1625: *A Rod for Run-awayes* (1625), *London Looke Backe* (1630) and *The Blacke Rod* (1630) (Dekker 1625, 1630a, 1630b; Wilson 1925).

Our second author, Nathaniel Hodges (1629–88), was a physician established in Walbrook Ward in the centre of the City. Born in the parish of Kensington, where his father was the vicar, he graduated from Oxford in 1659 (doctor of medicine) and settled in London, being admitted as a member of the College of Physicians the same year. Hodges was one of the very rare doctors to remain in London throughout the plague of 1665, treating patients at his practice and visiting them in their homes. The City of London rewarded him for his courage and dedication, making him its stipendiary physician. In May 1666, he published a first account of the plague, which was, in effect, only considerations of the symptoms and the cure of the disease (Hodges [1666] 1721: 16–35). In 1671, he gave a second account, this time providing details and analyses of the visitation in London: *Loimologia*[...] (Hodges 1671), which met with some success and for which the College of Physicians elected him a fellow the following year. Despite the recognition of the municipal authorities and his peers, Hodges fell into poverty and was sent to Ludgate Prison for debt. He died there in June 1688 (Stephen and Lee 1885–1900, vol. 27). *Loimologia* was translated into English and published in 1720 by John Quincy, a London apothecary (Hodges 1720).

The Wonderfull Yeare was published anonymously in 1603 (Thomas Dekker acknowledged the authorship three years later in *The Seven Deadly Sinnes*), and focuses on what Dekker considered to be the three 'wonders' of the year: the death of Elizabeth I, the accession of James I and the plague.[1] The latter occupies nearly two-thirds of the pamphlet, a testimony to the importance Dekker gave to the epidemic, which:

> in the Appenine height of this immoderate joy and securitie [accession of James I] (that like Powles Stéeple ouer-lookt the whole Citie [a reference to the steeple of St. Paul's Cathedral which was topped by the tallest spire in London. It was destroyed by fire in 1561 and never rebuilt]) Behold, that miracle-worker, who in one minute turnd our generall mourning to a generall mirth [accession of James I and death of Elizabeth I], does now againe in a moment alter that gladnes to shrikes & lamentation.
> (Dekker [1603] 1884: 102)

Dekker does not give an account of the plague as such; there is no attempt to set it within a timeframe, to look for its causes, to quantify the deaths (though he does state that there were more than 40,000: 'you the ghosts of those more (by many) then 40000, that with the virulent poison of infection have been driven out of your earthly dwellings', Dekker [1603] 1884: 103) or to detail measures taken (if any). In that respect, *The Wonderfull Yeare* does not inform the reader of the specificities of the visitation in London. But that was not Dekker's aim. He was writing a pamphlet to earn the living he could no longer make with the theatres closed. It had to sell and, as a (play)writer, Dekker knew very well how to keep his readers' interest high and not to bore them with dates and numbers for, as he wrote, 'But to chronicle these [the deaths] would weary a second *Fabian*' (Dekker [1603] 1884: 118), referring to Robert Fabyan's (sheriff of London in 1493, d. 1513) *Newe cronycles of Englande and Fraunce* (Fabyan 1516), which enjoyed many reprints in the sixteenth century under different titles.

Thus, *The Wonderfull Yeare* offers another type of discourse on the plague. It speaks directly to the Londoners, referring to churches and places (St. Paul's

Cathedral, Gravesend, Smithfield, Cheapside, St. Bartholomew Hospital, Bucklersbury, Bedlam, St. Gilles, St. Sepulchre, St. Olave, St. Clement, Birchin Lane, Stepney, London Bridge, the Thames, St. Mary Overie), sounds ('to hear the sound of Bow-bell till next Christmas' – a reference to the peal of bells of St. Mary-le-Bow Cheapside, which, as from 1472, were rung every night at 9; from 1520 a large bell sounded the end of work, Weinreb and Hibbert [1983] 1987: 80) and trades ('the strength of English Béere' – London enjoyed a reputation for good beer and there were several breweries in the City, the Brewers' Company being one of the oldest of the City guilds (Weinreb and Hibbert [1983] 1987: 84–86)); 'if one newe suite of Sackcloth had béene but knowne to have come out of Buchin-lane (being the common Wardrope for all their Clowneships)'; Birchin Lane was known for men's ready-made clothes shops (Weinreb and Hibbert [1983] 1987: 66) so familiar to them (Dekker [1603] 1884, respectively: 102, 111–14, 116, 121–22, 135, 138, 146, 148; 122; 116). Dekker compares the plague-ridden London to a 'dangerous sore Citie' that at night becomes a 'vast silent Charnell-house [...] hung (to make it more hideous) with lamps dimly & slowly burning, in hollow and glimmering corners' where 'many poore wretches, that in fieldes, in ditches, in common Cages, and under stalls [...] have most miserably perished' (Dekker [1603] 1884, respectively: 115; 104; 118). He tells of the infected houses being closed by order and their doors marked with the 'fatall hand-writing of death' and the drama unfolding behind: 'how often hath the amazed husband waking, found the comfort of his bedde lying breathlesse by his side! his children at the same instant gasping for life! and his servants mortally wounded at the hart by sicknes!' (Dekker [1603] 1884: 106).

The 1603 book of *Plague Orders* devotes a long paragraph to the necessity and importance of marking the infected houses:

> The houses of such persons out of the which there shall die any of the plague, being so certified by the viewers, or otherwise knowen, or where it shall bee understood, that any person remaineth sicke of the plague, to be closed up on all parts during the time of restraint, viz. sixe weeks, after the sicknesse be ceased in the same house, in case the said houses so infected shall be within any Towne having houses neere adjoyning to the same [...] and furthermore, some speciall marke shall be made and fixed to the doores of every of the infected houses.
>
> (Anon. 1603: paragraph 5)

He tells of the 'still and melancholy streets' their pavements covered, no longer with 'gréene rushes' but 'strewede with blasted Rosemary: withered Hyacinthes, fatall Cipresse and Ewe, thickly mingled with heapes of dead men bones' (Dekker [1603] 1884: 104–05). Dekker remarks on this 'strange alteration' brought on by the plague, as it was common practice in London to cover the streets with rushes for a funeral to hush the noise of the procession; rosemary was generally only used at a funeral to conceal the smell of putrefaction and was mostly associated with weddings (see Gittings 1984: 110–11): 'the rosemary that was washt in swéete water to set out he Bridall, is now wet in tears to furnish her buriall' (Dekker [1603] 1884: 129). Dekker notes that this sudden rise in the consumption of rosemary had pushed its price up: 'the price of flowers, Hearbes and garlands, rose wonderfully, in so much that Rosemary which had wont to be sold for 12. pence an armfull, went now for six shillings a handfull' (Dekker [1603] 1884: 114). If London was a 'dangerous sore Citie' it was also in a state of 'pittifull (or rather pittilesse) perplexitie [...], forsaken like a Lover, forlorne like a widow, and disarmed of all comfort'. Dekker also remarks, on several occasions, on the great numbers of deaths that transform the City into a '*Mare mortuum*': '40000 [...] heapes of dead mens bones [...] a thousand Coarses [...] dead Marches were made of thrée thousand trooping together' (Dekker [1603] 1884, respectively: 114; 109, 103–04, 112).

He describes – with the necessary exaggeration to emphasize the abnormality of the situation – the scenes of horror and desolation on many streets of the City:

> a thousand Coarses, some standing bolt upright in their knotted winding shéetes: others half moulded in rotten coffins, that should suddenly yawne wide open, filling his nosthrils with noysomestench, and his eyes with the sight of nothing but crawling wormes.
> (Dekker [1603] 1884: 104)

He tells of the noise that, during the day, accompanies the plague:

> the loud grones of raving sickemen [...] In every house [...] Servants crying out for maisters: wives for husbands, parents for children, children for their mothers[...] Bells heavily tolling in one place, and ringing out in another.
> (Dekker [1603] 1884: 105)

He makes clear that he believes the plague started in the 'sinfully-polluted Suburbes' and summons the image of war ('this mortalland pestiferous battaile') to explain the progression of the plague to the City. Death, personified as a Spanish Leaguer or Tamberlaine (a leaguer was a besieger and Tamberlaine is not only a reference to the Asian emperor Timur (d. 1455) but also to Christopher Marlowe's play *The Great Tamburlaine* written in 1587–88 and published in 1590 (Marlowe 1590)), having 'pitcht his tents, (being nothing but a heape of winding shéetes tackt together)' besieges London, whilst the plague is the 'Marshall of the field', its manifestations ('Burning Feavers, Boyles, Blaines, and Carbunclers') his officers, and the troops a mixture of 'dumpish

Mourners, merry Sextons, hungry Coffin-sellers, scrubing Bearers, and nastie Grave-makers' who acted as pioneers, 'Feare and Trembling' being the 'two Catchpolles of Death', those who arrested everyone. When the plague finally entered London, it behaved like an army let loose to freely kill, rape and ransack: 'this Invader [...] plaide the tyrant [...] Men, women & children dropt downe before him: houses were rifled, stréeetes ransackt, beautifull maidens throwne on their beds, and ravisht by sicknes' (Dekker [1603] 1884: 110–12. A catchpole was a sheriff's officer who arrested debtors, a figure familiar to many Londoners).

To his fellow citizens, Dekker pledges to put his craft and tools at their service to be the recorder of their sufferings: 'let me behold your ghastly vizages, that my paper may receive their true pictures: *Eccho* forth your grones through the hollow truncke of my pen, and raine downe your gummy teares into my Incke' (Dekker [1603] 1884: 103–04).

> He shares with them the fear, pain and misery that plague – the 'dreadfull a fellow', the 'ruffianly swaggerer' – provokes, and finds the words and images to express what all feel: 'A stiffe and fréezing horror sucks up the rivers of my blood: my haire stands an ende with the panting of my braines: mine eye balls are ready to start out, being beaten with the billowes of my teares'.
>
> (Dekker [1603] 1884: 102)

He laments the 'husbands, wives & children being led as ordinarily to one grave, as if they had gone to one bed' (Dekker [1603] 1884: 112). He sympathizes with those no longer safe in their own homes:

> death, like a thief, sets upon men in the hie way, dogs them into their own houses, breakes into their bed chambers by night, assaults them by day, and yet no law can take hold of him: he devoures man and wife: offers violence to their faire daughters: kils their youthfull sonnes, and deceives them of their servants.
>
> (Dekker [1603] 1884: 126)

He commiserates with wives and mothers who have lost loved ones: 'you desolate hand-wringing widowes that beate your bosomes over your departing husbands: you wofully distracted mothers [...] lye kissing the insensible cold lips of your breathlesse Infants' (Dekker [1603] 1884: 103).

Born in London and having experienced the hardships of life when money is scarce, Dekker understood the contempt and, no doubt, the resentment those – the poor – who could not flee the City, felt towards the rich inhabitants. He describes them abandoning their 'severall lodgings very delicately furnisht' and fleeing London to their 'Parkes and Pallaces in the Country', taking with them their earthly goods 'lading thy asses and their mules with thy gold (thy god), thy plate, and thy Iewels', leaving 'not a good horse in Smith-field, nor a Coach to be set eye on' (Dekker [1603] 1884: 106–07, 111). He blames the flight of the rich (that he calls 'runawayes' and cowards) for the quick fall of London to the plague's armies ('for the enemie taking advantage by their flight') and for the lack of charitable assistance for the poor ('*Lazarus* lay groning at every mans doore: mary no *Dives* was within to send him a crum'), and opposes the selfishness of the rich to the generosity of the poor, taking as an example the cobbler of a tale he tells his readers ('he sat distributing amongst the poore, to some, halfe-penny péeces, penny péeces to some, and two-penny péeces to others') (Dekker [1603] 1884: 111–12, 130). Dives stands for a very rich man. Dekker plays on the reference to the biblical parable of the rich man and Lazarus (Luke 16: 19–31) known to all his readers). He also opposes the conditions in which those who remained were buried ('rotten coffins', mass graves) to those reserved for the rich ('the everlasting brest of Marble'). But to console his poor reader, Dekker draws on the well-known image of the medieval *Dance of Death*, in which death leads by the hand rich and poor to their demise, regardless of their social status or their wealth.

The theme was well known to Londoners. A *Dance of Death* had been painted on the walls of the north cloister at St. Paul's Cathedral in the mid-fifteenth century. Though the Duke of Somerset (*c*.1550–52), the Lord Protector of England, had the cloister pulled down to give place to a garden in 1549, the *Dance* survived in manuscript and soon in print. John Lydgate (*c*.1370–*c*.1451) had translated the French *Danse Macabre* he had seen in Paris, in the Cimetière des Innocents, in 1422 and the manuscript was published (with woodcuts and additions) by Richard Tottel in 1544 at the end of John Lydgate's *The Fall of Princes* (*The Daunce of Machabree*, in Lydgate [1544] 1924–27: vol. 4, 1025–44). Londoners could also find reference to the *Dance* in Stow's *Survay of London*, which was first published in 1598 and reprinted in 1603 by John Windet with some additions (Stow [1603] 1908: vol. 1, 327–28). Dekker told his readers that flying to their 'Parks and Pallaces' had not saved the rich, as death had caught up with them and was as merciless in the country as it was in the City: 'the broad Arrow of Death, flies there up & downe, as swiftly as it doth here: they that rode on the lustiest geldings could not out-gallop the Plague' (Dekker [1603] 1884: 115). Despite being 'pampered with superfluous fare, so perfumed and bathed in odoriferous waters, and so gaily apparelled in varietie of fashions' (Dekker [1603] 1884: 107), dead, the powerful will be thrown, like paupers, into 'a rank & rotten grave [...] a mucke-pit' without any consideration or respect for their past glory. No doubt to please his reader and play on their feelings of revenge, but maybe also partly on account of experience, Dekker claims that the rich were badly received in the country ('the Country round about thée shun thée') where 'thy pride is disdained' and were refused burial in 'Church, or common place of buriall' where they could 'maintaine the memory of thy childe, in the everlasting brest of Marble' and had to dig the graves themselves (Dekker [1603] 1884: 108–09).

Dekker is very critical of the doctors, not only for their absence ('they hid their Synodicall heads aswell as the prowdest') but even more so for their incompetence – they were 'at their wits end' unable '(with all their cunning in their budgets) [to] make pursenets to take him [the plague] napping' – and for their incapacity to save lives. He ridicules their remedies, which consisted of a mixture of drugs ('Losinges, and Electuaries, Diacatholicons, Diacodiens [...] Antidotes'), medical practices ('Phlebotomies') and superstition ('Amulets') that 'turned to Durt' and 'their simples [which] were simple things' and are unable 'to hold life and soule together' (Dekker [1603] 1884: 116–17. A purse net was a special type of net used to catch fish or small animals; a diacatholicon was a purgative electuary (a powder or paste mixed with something sweet); a diacodien was an herbal remedy used to aid sleep). Dekker was only echoing his contemporaries' opinions of physicians and apothecaries and of their discourse on how to combat plague. Since the 1347–50 Black Death, many treatises were written, first in Latin, and then in vernacular languages to be more accessible, often drawing from the same author or borrowing from each other. Thus, the first book on the plague in English was a translation of Joannes Jacobi's (d. 1384) work of 1376, *De pestilencia*; it was published in 1485. Johannes Jacobi (or Jean Jacme) was professor of medicine at the University of Montpellier (France). *The De pestilencia* has been wrongly attributed to Benedictus Canuti (d. 1462). There are at least two editions of Jacobi's 'little book' in 1485 under two different titles, both published in London by William de Machlinia: *Here begynneth a litil boke the whiche traytied and reherced many godet hinges necessaries for the infirmite & grete sekenesse call pestilence: the whiche often times enfecteth us* (Jacobi 1485a) and *A passing gode lityll boke necessarye [and] behouefull a[g]enst the pestilence* (Jacobi 1485b). It enjoyed reprints, with slightly different titles, in 1509, 1520 and 1536. In 1603, Thomas Lodge published *A Treatise of the Plague* (Lodge 1603), which was a word-for-word translation of François Valleriole's *Traicté de la Peste* published in Lyon in 1566 (Cuvelier 1968; Valleriole 1566). Paul Slack estimates that there were 153 different books on medicine written in English between 1485 and 1604, 23 being exclusively concerned with plague. He also notes the increase in the number of religious tracts and sermons on plague in the seventeenth century. For example, in 1603–04, 28 books dealing with plague were published, of which fifteen were of a religious character (Slack [1985] 1990: 23–24). Nevertheless, since the debate in 1348 between Ibn Khatima (*c.*1324–69) who, in Almeria, believed that no cure was possible without the patient showing remorse and promising to live a righteous life and that plague was not contagious, and Ibn Al-Khatib (1313–74) who, in Granada, thought that the only way of containing plague was to break the chain of contagion, little progress had been made (Clément 2020: 12. See also Biraben 1975 and 1976). Dekker alludes to the belief that plague was sent by God: 'seeing the black & blew stripes of the plague sticking on his flesh, which he received as tokens (from heaven)' (Dekker [1603] 1884: 119). As Véronique Montagne points out, all these 'scientific' texts tended to cause anguish rather than reassure (Montagne 2010: 110).

Finally, in the second half of his pamphlet (pp. 126–48), Dekker regales his readers with several tragicomic stories, bringing laughter to pain and despair: that of young man deprived of possessing his young bride as she was struck by plague at their wedding, leaving her husband 'a widower, [who] never knew is wife'; that of the poor cobbler whose wife, dying of plague, admitted to him that she had cheated him ('had planted a monstrous paire of invisible hornes'); that of the drunkard (a 'worshipper of *Bacchus*') so drunk that he fell into an open grave thinking it was his bed; that of the fat rich Londoner seeking refuge in the country, falling dead in an inn and being buried naked in a field by a 'Tinker'; that of a country Justice of Peace who, for fear of catching the plague, refused to deal with some Londoners who had stolen a few apples in an orchard. All of these characters were recognizable by Londoners and related to well-known popular tales. Maybe Dekker thought that comic, ridicule and grotesqueness would help to alleviate his readers' sufferings, but, as a playwright, he also knew that making them laugh was an excellent selling factor for his pamphlet.

Loimologia (the study of pestilential diseases and plagues) is a very different book. Written by a doctor seven years after the plague, it has a more clinical approach to the subject and does not convey the same sense of intimacy with the sufferings of the Londoners, nor does it play on the pathos of the situation. Hodges claims that 'it is my Business here to adhere to Facts' (Hodges 1720: 6). Writing after the visitation, Hodges can recall the rapid return to life in the following months as soon as the plague receded: trade resumed, people socialized, marriages were celebrated, births increased (Hodges 1720: 27–28). In that respect, ending on a very positive note ('the People again chearfully went about'), as if the visitation had only been a sad parenthesis for the Londoners, *Loimologia* does not convey the intense sense of gloom and despair that runs through *The Wonderfull Yeare*. Nevertheless, it does share some themes with Dekker's pamphlet. The most striking are the personification of plague – depicted as an enemy ('devouring', 'cruel'), a 'cruel Destroyer' that 'reigned over whole Counties', '*Hydra's* Heads', a cruel midwife that made 'all Children, and Infants passed immediately from the Womb to the Grave' – (Hodges 1720: 14, 16), and the image of war waged by plague on the 'Soldiery' (Londoners). Hodges describes the disease rampaging through London in a 'running sort of Fight', writes of a 'redoubled Fury' and compares the way in which plague spread as not unlike what is often seen in Battle, when after some Skirmishes of Wings, and separate Parties, the main Bodies come to engage; so did this Contagion at first only scatter about its Arrows, but at last covered the whole City with Death' turning London into a 'Field of Death'.

(Hodges 1720: 12, 18)

According to Hodges, doctors were the only ones who knew 'in what Parts to attack the Enemy [and] with what Weapons to do it'. Hodges also draws on the same popular images as Dekker: that of death striking the newly married couple ('the Marriage-Bed changed the first Night into a Sepulchre, and the unhappy Pair meet with Death in their first Embraces') and that of the drunken man (Hodges 1720: 24, 16). As with Dekker, he is impressed by the noise of death, that of the dying: 'dying Groans [...], Ravings of a Delirium [...], not far off Relations and Friends bewailing':, and that of the bells ringing unceasingly: 'the Bells seemed hoarse with continual tolling' (Hodges 1720: 16, 18). He also summons the image of the *Dance of Death*:

> this Plague spare no Order, Age, or Sex; The Divine was taken in the very Exercise of his priestly Office, to be enrolled amongst the Saints Above; and some Physicians [...] could not find Assistance in their own Antidotes [...], many [died] in their old Age, others in their Prime [...] of the Female sex most died; and hardly any Children escaped.
>
> (Hodges 1720: 18)

He describes the same scenes of desolation: people staggering 'like drunken Men' in the streets and suddenly collapsing and dying, others lying 'vomiting as if they had drank Poison', and 'the burying Places [which] would not hold the Dead, but they were thrown into large Pits dug in waste Grounds, in Heaps, thirty or forty together' (Hodges 1720: 16–18).

As one could expect, Hodges does not complain of his fellow physicians. He praises their dedication and courage, remarking that eight or nine died caring for the sick, and proudly notes that even some 'very great and worthy Persons [...] voluntarily contributed their assistance in this dangerous Work', amongst whom he names the leading physicians and anatomists of the day: Peter Barwick (1619–1705), Humphrey Brooke (1617–93), Francis Glisson (1597–1677), Nathan Paget (1615–79) and Thomas Wharton (1614–73) (Hodges 1720: 14–15). On the other hand, he is extremely dismissive of nurses ('they are not to be mention'd but in the most bitter Terms'), accusing them of killing their patients by strangulation or by infecting them with the plague and then robbing them. It is unclear what proof Hodges had of their murderous business, as he admits that 'they were without Witnesses', or why he held nurses in such contempt (Hodges 1720: 8–9). He is also very critical of all those who were not physicians but nevertheless distributed or sold medicine, amongst whom he counts chemists ('Chymists'). Hodges has harsh words for these 'Quacks', 'Strangers to all Learning as well as Physick, [who] thrust into every Hand some Trash or other under the Disguise of a pompous Title'. He blames them for many a death, claiming that 'Their Medicines were more fatal than the Plague'. He bitterly regrets that the government allowed some unknown French remedy to be tried out on English patients on the basis that an English ambassador in Paris ('a Person of Distinction and great Humanity') had heard that 'some Frenchmen were Masters of an Anti-pestilential Remedy'); unfortunately – and as expected? – the *Mountain brought forth Death* (Hodges 1720: 21–23).

The real novelty of *Loimologia* lies in two areas. Firstly, Hodges attempts to chart the origin and progress of the plague. He states that it started at the end of 1664, in Westminster, where a family showed symptoms of the disease. It was spread to London by neighbours of the infected who sought refuge there. From then on, it became unstoppable. Hodges explains that, at first, the contagion was slowed down by a three-month hard frost during the winter (December onwards), but as soon as the weather improved, it 'gained Ground'. It increased 'through May and June, with more or less Severity; sometimes raging in one Part, and then in another', before returning with 'redoubled Fury'; Hodges notes that 8,000 people died in the space of a week, though does not give any precise date. The situation was particularly dramatic during August and September, when plague 'made a most terrible Slaughter, so that three, four, or five Thousand died in a Week, and once eight Thousand'. Hodges writes that the peak came in early September, when 'more than twelve Thousand died in a Week'. He also remarks that, during the summer, the disease rapidly took over the surrounding counties, carried by those who, in great numbers, had fled the City, and that the towns along the Thames were more severely hit because of the goods being shipped up and down the river. Plague then declined by 'leisurely Degrees' though did not vanish, whilst other diseases reappeared ('*Inflammations, Head-achs, Quinseys, Dysenteries, Small-Pox, Measles, Fevers,* and *Hectics*'). He remarks, not without a certain pride, that in the spring of 1666, a final bout of plague was quickly contained by the doctors (Hodges 1720: 1–2, 5–6, 11–12, 16, 19, 25–28). Hodges' chronology of the visitation tallies with other sources, and the number of deaths he gives for August and September are very similar to those calculated by Charles Creighton from the bills of mortality, except for the peak of 12,000, which is much higher than the 8,200–8,300 at which Creighton arrives (Creighton 1891: 662). Similarly, he estimates the number of deaths due to the 'Contagion' at 'about one hundred thousand', which corresponds approximatively to the total number of deaths for 1665 but is higher than those due to plague, according to Creighton (Hodges 1720: 28; see *supra*). Nevertheless, *Loimologia* remains a very accurate account of the development of the plague in London in 1665.

The second innovative aspect of *Loimologia* is that Hodges describes and comments on the measures taken by the government and the municipal authorities in their attempt to stem and eradicate the disease and the responses of the population and tries to give a 'scientific' explanation of the visitation (Anon. 1665b, 1721a). Three measures particularly interested him. The first was the order to lock up the entire household for 40 days as soon as symptoms of plague appeared in the house, to paint a red cross on the door with 'Lord have mercy upon us' inscribed underneath and to station a guard outside the house to deter anyone from leaving or entering and handing food and medicine to the interned. Hodges thoroughly disagrees with the practice, which he considers 'abhorent to Religion and Humanity' and contrary to 'that Liberty which is necessary for the Comforts both of Body and Mind'. He claims that it did not stop the plague, as locking 'sick and well together' increased mortality, that the quarantine was too strictly enforced and that it led neighbours to leave instead of helping the afflicted. Hodges suggests that when a house gets infected, separate lodgings should be provided for the sick in the City and for the healthy in the suburbs as 'the infected Breath poisons upon the healthful'. The second measure he disapproves of is the order to light fires in the streets of London for three days. Hodges says that his fellow physicians all thought that this could not have any effect because it was not the air that was infected. Ironically, the fires were washed out by heavy rain and the death toll increased. Finally, he totally condemns the authorization given for the sale of medicine by unqualified people, which endangered the population, causing more deaths ('the *Publick Health* also suffered') and regrets that the authorities did not listen to the advice the physicians tried to give them (Hodges 1720: 7–11, 19–20, 23–24). For Hodges,

> the fine Texture of a humane Body is not to be managed by [...] clumsie Hands [...] it is much better even to want Physicians in such Calamities, than to have the Sick under the Care and Management of the unlearned.
>
> (Hodges 1720: 24)

He dismisses all explanations that are not based on medical considerations or knowledge, though he does acknowledge their popularity amongst the 'common People'. He does not believe that there was any fatality or necessity that the plague should return every twenty years despite the regularity of previous visitations, the memories of which remained very vivid amongst Londoners ('terrified each other with Remembrances of a former Pestilence'). He also claims that the surge of plague had nothing to do with the 'Conjunctions of Stars, and the Appearances of Comets'. He blames those who fueled these popular beliefs of creating panic amongst the population, which help 'to propagate and inflame the Contagion', as the 'Populace' did not listen to 'Persons of Thought' (Hodges 1720: 3–5). In that respect, he greatly approved the decision taken by the government to ask the College of Physicians to devise a 'general Directory', written in English, for the conduct to be held and the measures to be imposed in case of plague (Anon. 1655a, 1721a). This was to replace the *Advice* appended to the *Orders*, which had not been updated since the late sixteenth century. He does not believe either that the visitation receded for lack of 'Subjects to act upon' (because of the number of deaths and of people who had fled), but that it followed a set pattern of slow rise and decline, and he notes that rather than stopping other diseases, it simply covered them up (Hodges 1720: 26). Nevertheless, despite his faith in medicine, Hodges does seem to believe that plague was sent by some divine providence, several times comparing the Great Plague of 1665 to the Great Fire of 1666. He lays responsibility for these 'two grievous Calamities' on a 'irresistable Fate' and suggests that plague, like fire, was a factor of regeneration and renewal for the City: 'the whole Malignity ceasing, the City returned to a perfect Health; not unlike what happened also after the last Conflagration, when a new City suddenly arose out of the Ashes of the old' (Hodges 1720: 2, 17–18, 26, 28).

Loimologia differs from the *Wonderfull Yeare* on an important point: it takes the viewpoint of the well-to-do, not that of the poor. Hodges does acknowledge that the plague brought great suffering ('The whole *British* Nation wept for the Miseries of her Metropolis [...] Even the Relation of this Calamity melts me into Tears') (Hodges 1720: 16, 19) and that the poor, who could not leave the City for lack of means to survive without work, were those the most affected and those who died in great numbers ('it is incredible to think how the Plague raged amongst the common People'), to the extent that the plague was called the '*Poors Plague*' (Hodges 1720: 15). He also acknowledges that the rich and powerful left London in haste and that the Court took refuge far away in Oxford ('the more opulent had left the Town, and it was almost left uninhabited'), but, unlike Dekker, Hodges never criticizes the rich for fleeing London. On the contrary, he claims that they greatly help the needy, thus alleviating their misery: 'their Necessities were relieved with a Profusion of good Things from the Wealthy [...] the beneficent Assistances of the Rich'. He also asserts that the municipal authorities were responsible for keeping markets open and prices of food low so that the poor were not left to starve and famine was avoided: 'by [...] the Care of the Magistrates; for the Markets being open as usual, and a greater Plenty of all Provisions, was a great Help to support the Sick; so that there was the Reverse of a Famine', and he actually blames the poor for overindulging in fruits: 'this Year was luxuriant in most Fruits, especially Cherries and Grapes, which were at so low a Price, that the common People surfeited with them' (Hodges 1720: 15, 19–21, 27).

The impression that Hodges does not consider himself to belong to the same (inferior) class is reinforced by the way in which he names the poor: 'common People', 'Populace', words that do not belong to the vocabulary of *The Wonderfull Yeare*.

Written 60 years apart, from two very different standpoints and at two different moments of the evolution of the disease, *The Wonderfull Yeare* and *Loimologia* are two complementary attempts to describe the impact of the visitation on London and its population. They capture the sufferings of those who could not – or did not want to – flee the City or the neighbouring parishes; the helplessness of the municipal authorities who were overwhelmed by the magnitude of the epidemic and left to cope with it, Court and Council having deserted in haste; the absence of any new cure, despite the regular recurrence of the visitation, but also the courage and abnegation of some. The only real novelty in over 60 years is the role played by the College of Physicians, officially asked in 1665 by the government to devise a new and more elaborate set of guidelines (*Directions*) for the population (Anon. 1655a, 1721a). Though this might have given some inhabitants the impression that more consideration was being bestowed upon a 'scientific' understanding and response to the plague, in reality, as Hodges angrily noted, the advice of the physicians – even of the most respected – was rarely taken into account. In very different words, Dekker and Hodges tell of the flight of the rich, the near abandonment of the poor and the exacerbation of the already acute class divide brought on by the plague, despite whatever help the rich were willing or forced to dispense. In that respect, *The Wonderfull Yeare* and *Loimologia* remain two invaluable firsthand accounts for understanding what plague meant in the seventeenth century.

NOTE

1. I am using here the reference 1884 edition by Alexander Grosart. *The Wonderfull Yeare* is at pages 73–148 and the account of the plague at pages 102–48.

REFERENCES

Anon. (1603), *Orders, Thought Meete by His Maiestie, and His Privie Counsell, to be Executed Throughout the Counties of This Realme, in Such Townes, Villages, and Other Places, as Are, Or May Be Hereafter Infected with the Plague, for the Stay of Further Increase of the*

Same. Also, an Advise Set Downe by the Best Learned in Physicke within This Realme, Containing Sundry Good Rules and Easie Medcines, without Charge to the Meaner Sort of People, Aswel for the Preservation of His Good Subiects from the Plague before Infection, as for the Curing and Ordering of Them after they Shalbe Infected, London: Robert Barker.

Anon. (1655a), *Certain Necessary Directions as Well for the Cure of the Plague, as for Preventing the Infection: With Many Easie Medicines of Small Charge, Very Profitable to His Majesties Subjects, Set Down by the College of Physicians*, London: John Bill and Christopher Barker [also in *A Collection of Very Valuable and Scarce Pieces Relating to the Last Plague in the Year 1665*, London: J. Roberts, 1721, pp. 36–52].

Anon. (1665b), *Rules and Orders to be Observed by All Justices of Peace, Mayors, Bailiffs, and Other Officers, for Prevention of the Spreading of the Infection of the Plague*, London: John Bill and Christopher Barker, 1665 [also in *A Collection of Very Valuable and Scarce Pieces Relating to the Last Plague in the Year 1665*, London: J. Roberts, 1721, pp. 1–12].

Anon. (1721a), *A Collection of Very Valuable and Scarce Pieces Relating to the Last Plague in the Year 1665*, London: J. Roberts.

Anon. (1721b), *Reflections on the Weekly Bills of Mortality, So Far as They Relate to all the Plagues Which Have Happened in London from the Year 1502, to the Great Plague in 1665, and Some Other Particular Diseases*, in *A Collection of Very Valuable and Scarce Pieces Relating to the Last Plague in the Year 1665*, London: J. Roberts, pp. 53–82.

Biraben, Jean-Noël (1975), *Les hommes et la peste en France et dans les pays européens et méditerranéens*, Paris and The Hague: Mouton.

Biraben, Jean-Noël (1976), *Les Hommes face à la peste*, Paris and The Hague: Mouton.

Clément, François (2020), 'A voir la légèreté de certains, on douterait des progrès accomplis depuis la peste noire', *Le Monde*, 23 March, p. 12.

Creighton, Charles (1891), *A History of Epidemics in Britain*, Cambridge: Cambridge University Press, 1891–1894, 2 vol., vol. 1: *From A.D. 664 to the Exctinction of Plague*.

Cuvelier, Elliane (1968), 'A treatise of the Plague de Thomas Lodge (1603): traduction d'un Ouvrage Medical Français', *Études Anglaises*, 21, pp. 385–403.

Defoe, Daniel (1722), *Journal of the Plague Year: Being Observations or Memorials of the Most Remarkable Occurrences, as Well Publick as Private, Which Happened in London during the Last Great Visitation in 1665*, London: E. Nutt, J. Roberts, A. Dedd, J. Graves.

Dekker, Thomas ([1603] 1884), The Wonderfull Yeare, in Alexander B. Grosart (ed.), *The Non-Dramatic Works of Thomas Dekker*, 5 vol., vol. 1, London and Aylesbury: Hazell, Watson and Viney, pp. 73–148.

Dekker, Thomas 1604a), *Nevves from Graves-end Sent to Nobody*, London: Thomas Creede.

Dekker, Thomas (1604b), *The Meeting of Gallants at an Ordinarie: or, the Walkes in Powles*, London: Thomas Creede.

Dekker, Thomas (1606), *The Seven Deadly Sins of London, Drawn in Seven Several Coaches, Through the Seven Several Gates of the City, Bringing the Plague with Them*, London: Nathaniell Butter.

Dekker, Thomas (1625), *A Rod for Run-awayes*, London: John Trundle.

Dekker, Thomas (1630a), *London Looke Backe at That Yeare of Yeares 1625: And Looke Forvvard, Vpon This Yeare 1630 Written Not to Terrifie, but to Comfort*, London: A. M.

Dekker, Thomas (1630b), *The Blacke Rod, and the Vvhite Rod (Justice and Mercie,) Striking, and Sparing*, London: B. A. and T. F.

Fabyan, Robert (1516), *Newe Cronycles of Englande and Fraunce*, London: R. Pynson.

Gittings, Clare (1984), *Death, Burial and the Individual in Early Modern England*, London: Croom Helm.

Green, Mary Anne Everett (ed.) (1857), *Calendar of State Papers, Domestic James I: 1603–1610*, London: Her Majesty's Stationary Office, 60 vol. Vol. 1: March–May 1603; vol. 2: June–July 1603.

Hodges, Nathaniel (1671), *Loimologia, Sive, Pestis Nuperae Apud Populum Londinensem Grassantis Narratio Historica*, London: Joseph Nevill.

Hodges, Nathaniel (1720), *Loimologia; or, an Historical Account of the Plague in London in 1665 ... To Which Is Added, An Essay on the Different Causes of Pestilential Diseases, and How They Become Contagious: With Remarks on the Infection Now in France and the Most Probable Means to Prevent It Spreading Here*. https://wellcomecollection.org/works/rxwns998. Accessed 03 June 2024.

Hodges, Nathaniel ([1666] 1721), *An Account of the First Rise, Progress, Symptoms, and Cure of the Plague: Being the Substance of a Letter from Dr Hodges to a Person of Quality*, London, Partly Reprinted in a Collection of Very Valuable and Scarce Pieces Relating to the Last Plague in the Year 1665, London: J. Roberts, pp. 13–35.

Jacobi, Johannes (1485a), *A Passing Gode Lityll Boke Necessarye [and] Behouefull A[g]enst the Pestilence*, London: William de Machlinia.

Jacobi, Johannes (1485b), *Here Begynneth a Litil Boke the Whiche Traytied and Reherced Many Godet Hinges Necessaries for the Infirmite & Grete Sekenesse Call Pestilence: The Whiche Often Times Enfecteth Us and a Passing Gode Lityll Boke Necessarye [and] Behouefull A[g]enst the Pestilence*, London: William de Machlinia.

Lodge, Thomas (1603), *A Treatise of the Plague: Containing the Nature, Signs, and Accident of the Same*, London: E. White and N. L.

Lydgate, John ([1544] 1924–27), *The Fall of Princes*, London: Richard Tottel. Reprinted with notes by Henry Bergen, *Lydgate's Fall of Princes*, London: Early English text Society (extra series, 121), 4 vol. *The Daunce of Machabree* is in vol. 4, pp. 1025–44.

Marlowe, Christopher (1590), *The Great Tamburlaine*, London: Richard Jones.

Montagne, Véronique (2010), 'Le discours Didascalique Sur la Peste Dans les Traités Médicaux de la Renaissance: Rationaliser et/ou Inquiéter', *Réforme, Humanisme, Renaissance*, 70, pp. 103–12.

Slack, Paul ([1985] 1990), *The Impact of Plague in Tudor and Stuart England*, Oxford: Clarendon Press.

Stephen, Leslie and Lee, Sidney (eds) (1885–1900), *Dictionary of National Biography*, London: Smith, Elder & Co., 63 vol.

Stow, John ([1603] 1908), *A Survay of London, Contayning the Originall, Antiquity, Increase, Moderne Estate, and Description of That Citie ... Also an Apologie (Or Defence) against the Opinion of Some Men, Concerning the Citie, the Greatnesse There Of. With an Appendix, Containing in Latine, 'Libellum De Situ & Nobilitate Londini', by W. Fitzstephen, in the Raigne of Henry the Second*, London: J. Windet. Edition with notes by Charles Letherbridge Kingsford, *A Survey of London by John Stow Reprinted from the Text of 1603*, Oxford: Clarendon Press, 2 vol.

Stow, John (1631), *Annales or a Generall Chronicle of England. Begun by John Stow: Continued and Augmented with Matters Forraigne and Domestique, Ancient and Modern, unto the End of this Present Yeere 1631, by Edmund Howes*, Gent., London: Richard Meighen.

Valleriole, François (1566), *Traicté de la Peste Composé Par Maistre François Valleriole Docteur en Medecine*, Lyon: Gryphius.

Weinreb, Ben and Hibbert, Christopher (eds) ([1983] 1987), *The London Encyclopaedia*, London: Macmillan.

Wilson, Frank P. (ed.) (1925), *The Plague Pamphlets of Thomas Dekker*, Oxford: Clarendon Press.

6

Representation of the Plague in Ancient Greek and Byzantine Texts and Responses to the COVID-19 Pandemic

Florian Steger

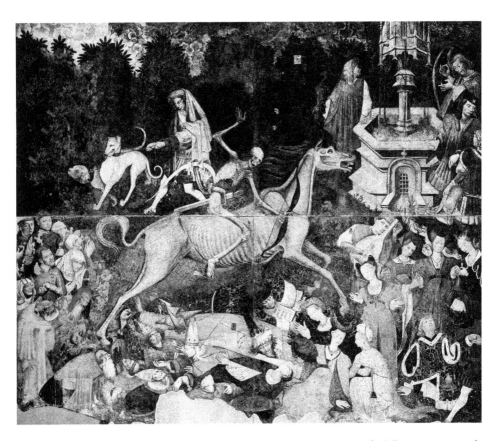

FIGURE 6.1: Unknown artist (possibly Guillaume Spicre), circa 1446. *Trionfo della Morte* (*Triumph of Death*). Originally in Palazzo Sclafani, now in Palermo's Regional Gallery, Palazzo Abatellis.

The god's arrows: The plague in Homer's Iliad

Throughout antiquity, a concept of health and disease in which the gods play a central role can be discerned in several cultural manifestations. This is why we speak here of a 'theurgic' concept of illness and health (Greek θεός: god, ἔργον: deed). In this framework, the process of healing, or even the ability to heal directly, is usually associated with individual deities, and sometimes also with heroic figures, who can cause or defeat illness through their superhuman attributes. The healing cult in ancient Greece focused on a few representatives, with Apollo, Asclepius and Hygieia as the central figures. Among the many diseases that can afflict people, 'plague' is also initially associated with a deity in ancient times – in this context, I use the word 'plague' to refer to highly infectious diseases with different mortality rates, regardless of their causative agent. Our earliest evidence is a well-known passage from Homer's *Iliad* (**T1**: Hom. Il. 1.42–53). In retaliation for a human offence, Apollo brings the λοιμός, the 'plague' to the Greeks by sending contaminated arrows into their camp. The word λοιμός is perhaps connected with λύμη ('outrage, maltreatment'), which could point towards the character of a personal punishment attributed to diseases sent by the gods. The reason for this punishment was the abduction of Chryseis, the daughter of Chryses, priest of Apollo, so that she could be given as a slave to the Greek army commander Agamemnon. Despite his attempt to get his daughter back by making counter-gifts to the Greeks, Chryses had been disrespectfully rejected by Agamemnon and therefore turned to Apollo for help. Only once the Greeks had appeased Apollo with ritual acts (i.e. cleansed themselves of their sins) did the god free them from the plague and restore their health.

The plague as a symbol of decadence: Thucydides' report

The theurgic conception of illness and health attested in the *Iliad* endured into late antiquity, mainly due to the sustained spread of the cult of the healing god Asclepius. Between the fifth and fourth centuries BCE, however, a rational medicine gradually developed that abandoned religious explanatory models and felt primarily committed to empirical observation. This is associated in the tradition with the figure of Hippocrates, of whom very little is actually known, and with the writings collected in the *Corpus Hippocraticum*.

The description of the Athenian plague handed down to us by the historian Thucydides (460/455–399/396 BCE) is clearly based on this new understanding of medicine. During the Peloponnesian War (431–404 BCE), the city-state of Athens was put in dire straits by the Peloponnesian power of Sparta. In his

History of the Peloponnesian War, Thucydides reports (Th. 2.47,3): 'Right at the beginning of summer, the Peloponnesians and their allies invaded Attica with two-thirds of their power, as they had done the first time [...] and devastated the country.'

In Thucydides' account, the invasion of Attica by the Peloponnesians is directly linked to the outbreak of the epidemic in Athens. Then a few months after the invasion, in 430 BCE, the plague put the *polis* of Athens to an additional hard test: 'They had not been many days in Attica when the plague broke out in Athens for the first time. [...] [N]owhere was such a plague, such a death of the people reported.'

The massive spread of an infection – to put it in modern terms – is here compared to an armed conflict taking place at the same time. Generally speaking, it can be said that language and images reminiscent of warlike conflicts are often used to describe infections. The plague broke out for the first time in the summer of 430 and continued until the summer of 428. It returned in the winter of 427/426 and then lasted until the winter of 426/425. It is extremely difficult to estimate the demographic consequences it had. Today, on the other hand, we are overwhelmed by data, we are almost conditioned to it. However, we often miss a critical approach here, as all data must be interpreted. Moreover, there is a dangerous potential in such seemingly exact numbers. This was impressively demonstrated again and again during the pandemic in countless discussions.

Inside the city of Athens, Thucydides says, not even the trained physicians could help. This is an image that has appeared again and again in epidemic history over the years when an overwhelming threat situation occurred and was often presented by the media in their portrayals of international conditions during the COVID-19 pandemic. And it is precisely the sudden occurrence of an unpredictable and completely new natural event that, in the current pandemic, has turned the initial uncertainty into the strength to seek new paths. Just think of the development of vaccines, which was extremely rapid, especially from the perspective of medical history – and in this respect, one should not be surprised if things are still sticking here and there. In this context, it is right to speak of a contingency of fate: We humans must recognize that nature has enormous penetrating power. And we would be well advised to put more resources into prevention.

In Athens, the epidemic was killing everyone. In the face of this hopeless situation and the deadly epidemic, there was neglect and immorality in society. What Thucydides describes can be interpreted as moral decay followed by political decay (Steger 2002, 2021: 482–83). Previously, Thucydides had Pericles sing the praises of the great power of Athens (2.35–46). The description of the epidemic represents a violent caesura. The historian describes the spread of the epidemic in Athens factually and clearly as an eyewitness and sufferer, connecting his description with the preventive goal of being prepared for future threats from epidemics (Th. 2.48,3):

> I will only describe how it was; only the characteristics by which one could most easily recognize it, in order to know if it should ever break out again, these I will describe, who myself was ill and saw others suffer.

History is written to remember; medical history is to provide for prevention. If we understand medical history not simply as a reservoir of solution options – which would certainly be too short-sighted – but as a complex, multi-faceted potential of experiences, it would indeed be worthwhile to look back for an understanding of today and tomorrow. This can be impressively demonstrated again and again, especially when dealing with infectious events.

Thucydides also describes the idea that there was a danger of infection from the sick, even for the animals (Th. 2.50,2). Especially endangered were those people who took care of the sick (T2 Th. 2.47,4):

> For the doctors were not only unable to treat the illness at first due to their lack of knowledge, but they were also dying in high numbers because they came into contact with it so much, and all other human skill was worth nothing.

As far as therapy was concerned, there was little to hand (Th. 2.51,3):

> Some died if they were left lying around, others died even with the best care. And no sure remedy was actually found that should have been used to help – what was useful to one was harmful to another – nor did any kind of body prove immune to it according to its strength or weakness, but it carried off all, even those who had lived so healthily.

The healthy were kept away from the sick, and only those who had already recovered – in modern terms we would say the immunized – dared to approach those affected. Sick people were abandoned and left alone with the disease (T2 Th. 2.51,6). Thucydides vividly describes the symptoms as in a medical treatise (T2 Th. 2.49,8). In this description, one is inevitably reminded of humoral pathology, i.e. of the first systematic theoretical efforts, collected in the writings of the *Hippocratic Corpus*, to assume natural explanations for the occurrence of illness, independently from the agency of gods (Craik 2001; Brodersen 2022). Thucydides is thus clearly influenced by the theories of contemporary medicine (Steger 2020: 60). According to these theories, a balance, an εὐκρασία, of the four humours (blood, phlegm, bile, and black bile) grants health, whereas the predominance of one of the humours, a δυσκρασία, leads to disease. In addition, there are primary qualities, such as moist, dry, cold, and hot, which correspond to the four humours. Based on these, certain therapeutic measures were then taken according to the principle *contraria contrariis curantur* ('opposites are healed by opposites'). So, if phlegm and thus the moist and cold predominated, warmth and dryness would be the therapeutic goal. And if there was too much blood and thus warmth and moistness dominated, dryness and coldness were the therapeutic goals – phytopharmaceuticals with corresponding effects were selected. In the case of infections, the breathing air of the sick person and air impurities, so-called *miasmata*, were considered possible sources of disease.

Byzantine representations of the plague

Existential threats from epidemics have been described throughout history for a long time. The so-called Justinian Plague, for example, spread pandemically across the entire Mediterranean region from 541 ADE onwards, lasted for two centuries and meant death for many people. Like Thucydides, the historiographer Procopius of Caesarea (*c*.500–560) experienced this event himself in Constantinople and expounded its effects in two chapters of his *De bello Persico* (T3 Procop. 2.22–23). If one closely follows Procopius' description, one will notice many parallels to the Thucydidean one, especially with regard to the psychosocial consequences (Whately 2017: 701).

The plague began in Pelusium, at the Nile Delta, and spread to southern Europe *via* Alexandria and Palestine – nevertheless, we can assume that its first origin is to be sought in Central Africa (Sarris 2007). In 542, it reached Byzantium. It manifested itself in fever and bubonic swellings. Once the first symptoms showed – Procopius tells us – the towns were quickly abandoned, and the dead were soon buried in mass graves due to lack of space. Physicians even resorted to the otherwise rarely practised dissection of corpses to determine the cause of the disease. Many wanted to see this as divine punishment for human sin – and so, help was also sought from God (Stathakopoulos 2007: 106–10; Horden 2005). Some still seek salvation today, then perhaps rather with the one God. As mentioned at the beginning, we speak here of theurgic models of illness: Gods send illnesses and gods can also bring about healings after reconciliation through offerings. Some people may be reminded of the pilgrimages to Lourdes and the miraculous healings that took place there.

The exact percentages of the epidemic's lethality cannot be established, although they are likely to be high (Rosen 2007: 209–10; Stathakopoulos 2007: 114–15). The epidemic's true impact as a catalyst for a change in Byzantine society is likewise disputed (Stathakopoulos 2007: 116–17).

The plague epidemic then returned in the fourteenth century – this is often referred to as the 'Black Death' (Vasold 1991: 38–93; Bergdolt 2017). It occurred in 1348/49 and came back in several waves until the Turkish conquest of Constantinople. It probably started in the Crimean harbour city of Kaffa (Wheelis 2002). The main report from a Byzantine perspective is provided by Emperor John VI Cantacuzenus (1295/96–1383) in his apologetic Ἱστορίαι (T4 Joh. Cant., Hist. 4.3; Bartsocas 1966). Because of its unusual features, he too interpreted the plague as a punishment from God. Cantacuzenus's description, like that of Procopius, stylistically resembles the model of Thucydides (Bartsocas 1966: 397–98; Miller 1976; Hunger 1976). We can find exact, sometimes literal, correspondences between Cantacuzenus and Thucydides in several locations; yet, despite its literary imitation, Cantacuzenus's account seems to remain faithful to an empirical assessment of the situation (Miller 1976: 393–94).

Quarantine measures were taken against infection. In 1374, this was first ordered in Reggio Emilia for ten days, in Ragusa (1377) and shortly afterwards since 1383 in Venice and Marseille – according to the term *quarantaine de jours* – for 40 days (Stathakopoulos 2016). The Italian author Giovanni Boccaccio describes this vividly in his *Decameron* (Wigand et al. 2020). The shipping routes were critically monitored. Ships with people suffering from the plague had to hoist a special flag and were not allowed to dock.

In the plague of 1348/49, protective clothing and plague masks with fragrant substances in their noses were therefore used. The idea that specific pathogens caused epidemics did not occur for a long time, even if, for example, the early modern physician Girolamo Fracastoro (1479–1553) took the right path with his idea of 'disease seeds'. More than two millennia passed before the plague could be effectively countered. In 1894, the Swiss biologist Alexandre Yersin discovered the plague pathogen named after him, the bacterium *Yersinia pestis* (Wagner et al. 2014). Subsequently, the chain of infection was described. Retrospective diagnostics should be treated with caution, as too little is known about the details and too much is based on today's view and terminology. The very use of the term 'plague' for the Attic plague is therefore not unproblematic, since it could easily lead to the conclusion that the plague around 430 was in fact the disease understood in this way today.

Responses to plague, ancient and modern

As we have seen so far, ancient and medieval sources that offer a representation of the unfolding of – and reactions to – epidemic diseases can be extremely helpful for a historically conscious assessment of the current pandemic situation. A common feature of historical descriptions of the plague is that reactions to epidemics are often ambivalent and contradictory, e.g. fear and withdrawal vs. joy and living for the moment, compassion and altruism vs. profit maximization, feelings of equality and solidarity as people from all social classes are affected vs. increased social inequalities once the sources dry up, and hope to survive vs. uncertainty and despair. Reactions to pandemics are complex and fluctuate between opposing positions in society and among individuals (Wigand et al. 2020).

As to the question of the cause of the epidemic, Thucydides wisely holds back (Th. 2.48,3):

> the opinion also arose that the Peloponnesians had thrown poison into the wells (for there was no spring water there at that time). Later it also reached the upper city, and there the people died more than ever. Now everyone may say about it, doctor or layman, what in his opinion was probably the origin of it and what causes he believes to have had an effect down to such depths; I will only describe how it was.

This is reminiscent of the medieval tradition of believing that Jews who poisoned wells were responsible for the plague, and once again it is reminiscent of modern discussions that lead to absurd and dangerous conspiracy theories. Anyone who witnessed our pandemic knows how many such absurd theories we had to endure. It is a frightening anthropological fact that we humans keep fuelling such conspiracy theories and thus perpetuate this unspeakable tradition. It would be much more effective to put all our energy into overcoming the pandemic as a gesture of solidarity.

The social consequences of the Athenian plague were depressing. Suddenly the splendour of the great power of Athens was tarnished. The plague came with the Spartans and initiated the decline (Th. 2.50,1): 'For the incomprehensible nature of the disease assailed everyone with a force beyond human measure.'

Athenian citizens were marked by despondency, despair and fear of infection (T2 Th. 2.51,4):

> The most terrible aspect of the disaster was the discouragement as soon as anyone realized they were sick (for they immediately turned to despair, thus giving themselves up to the thought too quickly and not making any resistance), and that each person while caring for another became infected and they died like sheep. It was thus that the majority of the deaths happened.

Keeping one's distance was already used as a proven means to avoid infection during the Attic disease. And this is remarkable since the commandment to keep at a distance remains the first choice in dealing with the current pandemic to this day. But at the same time, Athens lacked devotion and care for its neighbours. Only those who had recovered from the disease were willing to help. Immorality spread among the citizens, and the laws were disregarded (**T2** Th. 2.53,4):

> No fear of the gods, nor human law, persisted, but people recognized that they saw everyone dying the same, whether pious or not, and nobody expected his life to last long enough to receive justice for wrongdoing, or to pay any fines.

The moral decline had become unstoppable. And such a decline is also not unknown to us in view of the recent pandemic. Especially when looking at the consequences of this pandemic from a global perspective, frightening psychosocial consequences can be described. Here, we must not be deceived by a national perspective; rather, the global dimensions that the pandemic has are still too little discussed publicly.

In his work *Palliativgesellschaft*, the Korean German philosopher and historian of culture Byung-Chul Han (2020) puts forward the central thesis of a permanent anaesthetization of our society, i.e. a 'palliative' democracy that no longer seeks painful confrontation. This thesis can certainly be argued about. But when Han states the following about the consequences of the pandemic in the chapter *Ethik des Schmerzes*, one can only agree, and observe the proximity to Thucydides' observations:

> In times of pandemic, the suffering of others recedes even more into the distance. It dissolves into numbers of cases. People die alone in intensive care units, without any human attention. Proximity means contagion. Social distancing exacerbates the loss of empathy. It turns into mental distancing. The other person is now a possible carrier of the virus, from whom it is important to keep a distance. Social distancing becomes an act of social distinction.

Accordingly, in a Nursing Ethical Reflection on Measures for the Containment of COVID-19 (Pflegeethische Reflexion der Maßnahmen zur Eindämmung von Covid-19) by the German Academy for Ethics in Medicine (2020), it is pointed out that, on the part of nursing, physical presence is an enormously valuable asset. Social isolation and deprivation are addressed as dangers of social distancing. Dignified care for those in need of care is demanded in the area of conflict between the risk of infection, physical closeness and quality of life, i.e. physical, no social distancing.

This is all the more reason, therefore, to not leave anyone alone in times of a pandemic with COVID-19. Currently, we are resorting to the effective imperative of keeping our distance in order to contain the infection. In order to enforce this distance, justification and proportionality are required; after all, civil liberties are being restricted here, and this is not without public resistance. In his novel *The Plague*, Albert Camus describes how difficult it is to take this 'monstrous' step in the Algerian city of Oran in the 1940s with a long arc of tension that finally ends in the caesura-setting telegram: 'Declare state of plague, close city.'

And the momentous words follow just as calmly: 'It may be said that from that moment the plague affected us all [...] and it was impossible to take account of individual cases.'

Where this can lead is shown by current developments in Poland and Hungary (Orzechowski et al. 2021): civil liberties were severely restricted during the COVID-19 pandemic. It becomes clear how strongly such decisions are supported by political interests. Here, protection against infection quickly becomes an argument for political interests when fundamental rights are restricted. The stepmotherly neglected health system now becomes quite obvious in its desolate situation. Added to this is politically co-determined access to the health system, which remains closed to migrants, for example. But also in general, sick people and people in need of care in Germany received worse care during the first months of the pandemic. In the meantime, data are available that show that due to the implementation of politically imposed restrictive measures – at least in parts – adequate health care for sick people could no longer take place. This includes patients with cancer whose therapies were or could not be continued. Elective surgery was postponed, and chemo-, radio- and palliative therapy took place later or irregularly. Many operations were cancelled. The use of screening examinations during the pandemic is also a cause for concern. In addition, patients with cardiovascular diseases should be mentioned, some of whom were not treated at all or were treated too late for fear of infection. But even simple dental treatment was only carried out to a limited extent due to political decisions. Last but not least, one should also think of mental disorders that have newly appeared or have worsened during a restricted medical care offer. The consequences of this inadequate medical care are likely to be severe.

And yet, in modern civil society, the individual must be protected and valued in his or her individuality. Under no circumstances should people be set off against people. That would be a serious violation of our constitution. Even if resources are scarce, every human life is to be respected and valued in the same way qua being human. What this can lead to is shown by Thucydides and those Byzantine historians who later relied on his account.

ACKNOWLEDGEMENT
Many thanks to Dr Vincenzo Damiani, who provided excellent support as a research assistant.

Appendix

T1 Homer, *Iliad* 1.42–53 (own translation).
'May the Danaians pay for my tears by your arrows.'
So in his prayer he spoke, and Phoebus Apollo heard him.
He came down from the peaks of Olympus, raging in his heart.
Upon his shoulders he carried his bow and close-covered quiver.
The arrows clattered upon his shoulders
in his angry motion; he darted down like night.
There was a dreadful twang from the silver bow.
First he attacked the mules and swift-footed dogs
but then he began to shoot his piercing missiles
at the men. The crowded pyres burned constantly with the dead.
For nine days the shafts of the god poured down upon the army [...].

T2 Thucydides, *History of the Peloponnesian War* 2.47–53 (own translation).
The doctors were not only unable to treat the illness at first due to their lack of knowledge, but they were also dying in high numbers because they came into contact with it so much, and all other human skills were worth nothing. [...]. **48.** It is said that it began in Ethiopia beyond Egypt, and then came into Egypt and Libya and into a large part of the land of the king. It attacked the city of the Athenians suddenly, and first touched the people of the Piraeus, so that it was believed based on this that the Peloponnesians had thrown drugs into the wells. [...]. **49.** If anyone was already sick with any disease, it turned into this one. Others, for no reason, but having been perfectly healthy suddenly developed painful aches in their heads and red spots and inflammation in their eyes, and inside, their throats and tongues immediately became bloody and their breath became foul and evil-smelling. Next came sneezing and hoarseness, and soon the disease descended into the chest with a powerful cough. Once it settled upon the stomach, it caused it to be upset, and pour out every purgation of bile ever named by doctors, and this with great pain. Most were afflicted with empty retching, causing great spasms, after which some felt relief, but for others, this came only much later. The body, if touched from the outside, was not overly hot or pale, but it was reddish, livid and covered in small blisters and ulcers. But inside it burned so strongly that one could bear not even the cover of the thinnest clothes or linen blankets, or anything other than nakedness, and would gladly have plunged oneself into cold water. [...] **51.** The most terrible aspect of the disaster was the discouragement as soon as anyone realized they were sick (for they immediately turned to despair, thus giving themselves up to the thought too quickly and not making any resistance), and that each person while caring for another became infected and they died like sheep. It was thus that

the majority of the deaths happened. For either because of fear they avoided each other, and so died alone, and many houses became empty and there was nobody to care for the sick [...]. Those who had recovered particularly pitied the dying and sick, since they knew that they were now safe; for the disease did not take attack the same person a second time, at least not fatally. [...]. **52.** All the customs which had previously applied to burials were completely shaken up, and everyone just buried as well as he could. [...]. **53.** No fear of the gods, nor human law, persisted, but people recognized that they saw everyone dying the same, whether pious or not, and nobody expected his life to last long enough to receive justice for wrongdoing, or to pay any fines.

T3 Procopius, *Persian War* 2.22–23 (own translation).
22. However, there is no means of either naming or devising any reason for this misfortune, unless one ascribes it to God. [...] It (*sc.* the disease) began among the Egyptians who lived in Pelusion. Then it divided in two and travelled into Alexandria and the rest of Egypt, and on the other side into the part of Palestine that borders Egypt [...]. So at first those affected tried to ward it off by calling upon the most sacred names and performing other sacred rites, as each was able to, but they accomplished absolutely nothing, since the majority of those who sought refuge in the sanctuaries died. [...] The infection proceeded in the following way. They would fall ill with a sudden fever, some while sleeping, others while walking around or doing any kind of activity. The body did not differ from its previous complexion, and it was not hot, despite the attack of fever, and there was not even any inflammation, but instead the fever was so weak from the beginning until the evening that neither the patients themselves nor the attending doctor thought that there was any danger. For none of those infected seemed to die from it. On the same day for some, but the next day for others, or even a few days later, a swelling (*boubon*) would develop, not only on the part of the body which is below the abdomen, called the groin (*boubon*), but also in the armpit, and in some cases, it even occurred even next to the ears and in various parts of the thighs. Up to this point the progression was nearly the same for everyone infected by the disease. After this I cannot say whether the difference in symptoms was the result of different physical conditions of patients, or whether it progressed according to the will of the one who sent the disease. For some went into a deep sleep, while others experienced extreme delirium, though both groups suffered the symptoms peculiar to the disease. [...] In the cases when the patient neither fell asleep nor experienced delirium, the swelling became gangrened and they died in excruciating pain. [...] In their perplexity and ignorance of the symptoms, some doctors thought that the source of the disease must be found in the swellings, and they decided to examine the bodies of those who had died. They cut open some of the swellings and found

a dreadful kind of pustule which had developed inside. [...] **23.** When all the burial places which had existed before, were filled up with corpses, they dug up all the areas around the city, and they put the dead there, as far as possible, and they left them. [...] At that time it seemed that there was not a single healthy person to be seen in the markets in Byzantium, but everyone who happened to remain physically healthy sat at home, either caring for the sick or mourning the dead.

T4 Johannes Cantacuzenos, *Histories* 4.3 (own translation).
When she (*sc.* the empress Irene) came to Byzantium, she found Andronicus the younger of the sons had died of the plague that was raging at that time. It had started among the Hyperborean Scythians, before spreading across nearly the whole inhabited world and killing many of the inhabitants. [...] **50.** If anyone was already sick at all, their illness soon turned to this one, and no doctors' skill was sufficient, nor was it similar in all patients, but some were unable to hold out even a short time and died on the same day, others in a single hour. Those who resisted for two or three days first experienced severe fever, before the disease attacked the head [...]. But in other cases it did not attack the head: instead the illness attacked the lungs, and internal inflammation developed immediately, and produced sharp chest pains [...]. **51.** Throughout everything there was confusion on all sides. Upon the upper and lower arms abscesses developed. For some these were also on the jaws, and various patients had them on different parts of the body. Some had more, some less, and black bubbles erupted from them. [...] Of the many afflicted, the few who were able to recover were no longer vulnerable to the same illness, but were then safe. The disease did not attack a second time with fatal results [...]. The discouragement was the most terrible part. **52.** For whenever someone realized that he had become sick, there was no hope of recovery, but they despaired, let themselves go and died immediately, adding their discouragement to the disease's great strength. The nature of the disease was beyond description. It can only really be observed that it was not one of the natural and habitual trials humankind faces, but was something entirely different which was imposed upon humankind by God for the sake of moderation.

REFERENCES

Academy for Ethics in Medicine (2020), 'Pflegeethische Reflexion der Maßnahmen zur Eindämmung von Covid-19', Diskussionspapier der Akademie für Ethik in der Medizin, https://www.aem-online.de/fileadmin/user_upload/2020_05_12_Pflegeethische_Reflexion_Papier.pdf. Accessed 20 April 2022.

Bartsocas, Ch. S. (1966), 'Two fourteenth century Greek descriptions of the "Black Death"', *Journal of the History of Medicine and Allied Sciences*, 21:4, pp. 394–400.

Bergdolt, K. (2017), *Der Schwarze Tod. Die Große Pest und das Ende des Mittelalters*, München: C. H. Beck.

Brodersen, K. (ed.) (2022), *Hippokrates: Sämtliche Werke. Mit einer Einführung von Florian Steger*, Darmstadt: Wissenschaftliche Buchgesellschaft.

Craik, E. M. (2001), 'Thucydides on the plague: Physiology of flux and fixation', *Classical Quarterly*, 51, pp. 102–08.

Han, B.-Ch. (2020), *Palliativgesellschaft. Schmerz heute*, Berlin: Matthes & Seitz.

Horden, P. (2005), 'Mediterranean plague in the age of Justinian', in M. Maas (ed.), *The Cambridge Companion to the Age of Justinian*, Cambridge: Cambridge University Press, pp. 134–60.

Hunger, H. (1976), 'Thukydides bei Johannes Kantakuzenos. Beobachtungen zur Mimesis', *Jahrbuch der Österreichischen Byzantinistik*, 25, pp. 181–93.

Miller, T. S. (1976), 'The plague in John VI Cantacuzenus and Thucydides', *Greek, Roman and Byzantine Studies*, 18, pp. 385–95.

Orzechowski, M., Schochow, M. and Steger, F. (2021), 'Balancing public health and civil liberties in times of pandemic', *Journal of Public Health Policy*, 42, pp. 145–53.

Papadopoulos, A. (2019), 'Ένα αινιγματικό χωρίο στην Oratio funebris in Stylianam filiam του Μιχαήλ Ψελλού', *Зборник радова Византолошког института/Zbornik radova Vizantološkog instituta*, 56, pp. 95–107.

Rosen, W. (2007), *Justinian's Flea: Plague, Empire and the Birth of Europe*, London: Jonathan Cape.

Sarris, P. (2007), 'Bubonic plague in Byzantium: The evidence of non-literary sources', in L. K. Little (ed.), *Plague and the End of Antiquity. The Pandemic of 541–750*, Cambridge: Cambridge University Press, pp. 119–34.

Stathakopoulos, D. (2007), 'Crime and punishment: The plague in the Byzantine Empire, 541–749', in L. K. Little (ed.), *Plague and the End of Antiquity. The Pandemic of 541–750*, Cambridge: Cambridge University Press, pp. 99–118.

Stathakopoulos, D. (2016), 'Seuchen', in E. Kislinger (ed.), 'Medizin', in F. Daim (ed.), *Byzanz. Historisch-kulturwissenschaftliches Handbuch*, Stuttgart: J.B. Metzler, pp. 1039–46.

Steger, F. (2002), 'Herodots babylonischer Logos und die Seuche in Athen um 430 v. Chr', *Klio. Beiträge zur Alten Geschichte*, 84, pp. 27–36.

Steger, F. (2020), 'Ein wertvoller Blick in die Antike für Heute. Von der Attischen Seuche in Zeiten der Pandemie COVID-19', *Antike Welt. Zeitschrift für Archäologie und Kunstgeschichte*, 51:4, pp. 58–62.

Steger, F. (2021), *Antike Medizin. Einführung und Quellensammlung*, Stuttgart: Anton Hiersemann.

Vasold, M. (1991), *Pest, Not und schwere Plagen: Seuchen und Epidemien vom Mittelalter bis heute*, München: C. H. Beck.

Wagner, D. M. et al. (2014), 'Yersinia pestis and the Plague of Justinian 541–543 AD: A genomic analysis', *The Lancet Infectious Diseases*, 14:4, pp. 319–26.

Whately, C. (2017), 'Thucydides, Procopius, and the historians of the later Roman Empire', in S. Forsdyke, R. Baltot and E. Foster (eds), *The Oxford Handbook of Thucydides*, Oxford: Oxford University Press, pp. 692–707.

Wheelis, M. (2002), 'Biological warfare at the 1346 Siege of Caffa', *Emerging Infectious Diseases*, 8:9, pp. 971–75.

Wigand, M., Becker, Th. and Steger, F. (2020), 'Psychosocial reactions to plagues in the cultural history of medicine: A medical humanities approach', *The Journal of Nervous and Mental Disease*, 208, pp. 443–44.

7

'Let every man drinke in his own cup, and let none trust the breath of his brother': Encountering Plague in Early Modern Port Cities

James Brown and Gabrielle Robilliard

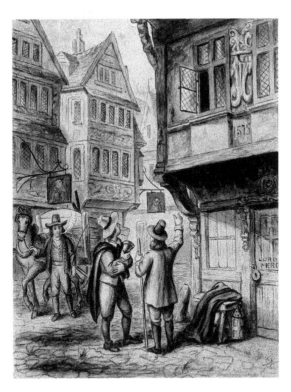

FIGURE 7.1: Cruikshank, George, *A cart for transporting the dead in London during the great plague* (1833), Watercolour painting. 18.5 × 14 cm. The Wellcome Collection. Courtesy of the Wellcome Collection ⓢ.

This engraving by the celebrated nineteenth-century illustrator George Cruikshank, commissioned for a Victorian edition of Daniel Defoe's 1722 classic *A Journal of the Plague Year*, offers a vivid dramatization of Londoners encountering the plague in 1665 (Evans and Evans 1978: 75). The last and most severe of seven such outbreaks that swept the seventeenth-century metropolis, it ravaged all but four of London's 130 parishes, killing an estimated 56,000 people in total, roughly an eighth of the population (Champion 1995). The image, based closely on Defoe's account, depicts three men with a horse and cart engaged in the grim errand of collecting the plague dead. They stand before an infected house that, in line with standard practice, has been padlocked and inscribed with crosses and divine invocations; one of the men smokes a pipe of tobacco, whilst in the background, the pictorial signboards of drinking houses hang forlornly. In its powerful conjoining of the ideas of pestilence, bodies (dead and alive), urban spaces, sociability and intoxicants, Cruikshank's grim retrospective vision nicely encapsulates and introduces the themes we will be exploring in this article.

As for our forebears, one of the most immediate impacts of the public health measures developed in response to the COVID-19 pandemic was on the urban environment. Local and national lockdowns caused pubs, cafés, restaurants and shops to close their doors or, at best, to resort to takeaway, delivery and click-and-collect, turning once bustling streetscapes into veritable ghost towns. Social distancing measures likewise reconfigured the way we used and interacted in many public spaces, guided by a shift away from pleasure to the perfunctory: we ventured out of houses only with purpose, diligently practised the pedestrian dodge and queued patiently for our daily necessities in well-spaced lines snaking down pavements. This enforced emptying of social spaces had a lasting impact, and we are still coming to grips with the long-term consequences of this prolonged sociability hiatus, which range from increased alcohol and drug abuse and higher incidence of depression to developmental issues amongst children and young people (Ornell et al. 2020; UNICEF Data Hub n.d.). Clearly, public spaces are essential to our individual and collective wellbeing because shared spaces are zones of social interaction and humans are social beings. But do all societies across time and space comprehend public spaces and react to phenomena that threaten these spaces in the same manner? If not, then how can we account for these differences? And finally, how can study of the past help us to reflect on tensions over spatial uses today?

As Cruikshank's etching makes clear, a useful historical analogue for these present-day crisis developments is the so-called second plague pandemic, a major series of outbreaks (starting with the Black Death of 1347–51) which visited death and devastation in European cities on a recurring basis between the fourteenth and eighteenth centuries. Historians have long approached these flare-ups from the perspective of public health, that is, they have sought to reconstruct and understand contemporary medical responses first and foremost. Therefore, attention has focused on the emergence of measures to combat the dire social and physical consequences of gruesomely sudden and high mortality: quarantine, isolation, dedicated plague hospitals, plague doctors and nurses, trading bans and so on (Slack 1988). Historical demographers sought to get a statistical handle on excess mortality during epidemics, making use of parish burial records and official mortality lists known in European cities by various names – bills of mortality in London, or books of the dead in Milan – that kept a public tally of death tolls (Benedictow 1987; Cohn and Alfani 2007). Others have pursued social, cultural and political approaches that explore, for example, how plague shaped a new relationship between the state and its subjects, functioning thus as a catalyst for the emergence of modern statehood (Dinges 1995; Dinges and Schlich 1995).

We take a different approach here, one that seeks to apprehend historical epidemics not merely as medical, demographic or political phenomena but also as socio-spatial ones. We want to examine them from the angle of urban public spaces because it was precisely these environments – the street, the tavern, the town square, the church – that were subject to so much governmental and medical circumscription during outbreaks. Drawing upon sources from four major ports in Northern Europe (Amsterdam, Hamburg, London and Stockholm), and inspired by the so-called spatial turn that has enhanced geographical sensitivities across the humanities and social sciences over the past three decades (Kümin and Usborne 2013), we will ask precisely what it meant to encounter plague in the early modern city, with special reference to urban surroundings and the sociability that unfolded within them in order to comprehend this logic of urban public spaces during times of plague, we have to first understand how contemporaries conceived of the disease. So, our first question is: what was plague?

Plague

The number of victims varied greatly from epidemic to epidemic, but – in stark contrast to COVID-19 – mortality rates were generally brutally high. London's 1603 contagion claimed the lives of around 17.8 per cent of the population and the 1665 outbreak – famously 'put out' for posterity by the Great Fire of London in 1666 – sent around 14 per cent of Londoners to their graves (Slack 1985: 144–64). Yet there was high variability between cities and epidemics, with the 1712/13 epidemic in Hamburg, for example, killing only around 10 per cent of inhabitants (Gernet 1869: 279).[1] Unlike many other kinds of contagion, plague did not usually recur every year or even every few years. The more frequent outbreaks of the late Middle Ages and Renaissance gave way in the second half of the seventeenth century to more prolonged intervals between epidemics. Some cities managed to avert fate for more than a generation; Hamburg, for example, experienced an outbreak between 1663 and 1665 but was spared the catastrophic epidemic that swept through Europe in the early 1680s and remained 'plague free' until 1712/13. But fortune notwithstanding, the ghoulish spectre of a scythe-wielding death was omnipresent, from the memento mori of decaying, fly-blown fruit portrayed in a fashionable still lives to the dancing skeletons of death adorning the walls and altars of baroque churches and in baroque visual culture (Mignon c.1670; University of Glasgow Library n.d.). Plague was as much a metaphorical danger to the community as it was an existential threat to bodies and souls; as Colin Jones argues, plague writings were about 'the myth of a personal, religious, and community life violated and inverted, plus the myth of salvation and integrity refound' (Jones 1996: 117). Plague ruptured community life, causing the cogs of the quotidian to grind to a halt, to be replaced by extraordinary orders placing bans on movement, trade and socializing. For those who could flee to the countryside – getting out was considered the most promising strategy for survival – leaving behind a town or city in a state of emergency and desperate for divine deliverance from moral and physical disorder.

For those unlucky enough to fall ill, a swift yet tortuous death was usually on the cards. In its bubonic form – that which caused large pus-filled swellings under the arms and in the groin, symptoms we most commonly associate with the historical disease today – plague killed between 60 and 80 per cent of its victims (Jones 1996: 100). The pneumonic form (affecting the lungs) was even more deadly. Death from both variants occurred within days and the illness spread rapidly, often wiping out entire households on the same day (Cohn and Alfani 2007: 203–04). In the face of such lethality, physicians often retreated into powerless humility: 'The Plague', the Amsterdam physician Paul Babette (1620–65) wrote, 'is a Disease whose nature is not to be comprehended by us' (Barbette 1687: 343). Physicians such as Hamburg's city physician Johann Bökel (1535–1605) knew that physic had no therapeutic answer to plague, but instead that 'in these dangerous times, it is preservation, and that one prevents the fever, before it begins, more than cure that is required' (Bökel 1597: Aiii [Vorrede], translation added). Once the sickness took hold and the patient was wracked by fever, thirst, vomiting and headache, followed by frenzy, painful buboes and a putrid stench issuing from the body, recovery was as much a matter of fate as for medical skill.

During the seventeenth and early eighteenth centuries, there was broad consensus amongst medical practitioners and writers that plague had to do with corruption of the air, commonly known as miasma. In 1597, Bökel described the air as 'polluted by evil mists and much dampness, or through watery vapours', or otherwise 'locked still, and does not move, so that it then tends towards foulness, and the less it moves, the fouler it becomes' (Bökel 1597: 32, translation added; Newman 2012). Other European commentators referred variously to 'venomous vapors', 'filthy savors', 'pestilential miasmata' or 'evil and unwholesome aire' (Kemp 1665: 15; Hodges 1720: 45). Hot weather was a harbinger of plague, generally a seasonal epidemic commencing in summer or autumn. Early modern people knew that the disease was transmissible, although, of course, they did not associate infection with a specific bacterium. Rather, plague was a slippery concept: it was just one expression of epidemic 'feverish illness' ubiquitous particularly during the summer and autumn months and its signs were many and varied. It was no straightforward matter to know when you were talking about *the* plague, as opposed to other feverish contagions. During the early eighteenth-century epidemic in Hamburg, for example, the city magistrates spent several months successfully denying claims that plague was in the city even though larger numbers of people than usual were dying in feverish, epidemic-like circumstances (Boyens 2004: 302–05).

Early modern medical theory considered plague to be transmitted variously through breath, via the skin, sweat or vapours. Fevered, infected bodies were thought to emit a 'contagious and poisonous Atmosphere' that could infect persons nearby (Quincy 1721: 51). Soft and absorbent materials and objects that had come into contact with infected persons or came from infected places were also thought to 'catch' the 'poison' and pass it on. Used and new bedding, clothing, paper and fabrics such as cotton, linen and wool were considered particularly dangerous and were subject to lengthy quarantine and disinfection before reuse or entry into the marketplace.

Bodies

These theories of plague causation and transmission were underpinned by an understanding of health, ill health and body based upon Galen of Pergamum's (129–216 CE) humoral theory, which was grounded in a particular relationship between the microcosm (the body) and the macrocosm (the outside world). According to Galenic theory, the body consisted of four humours and it was permeable and constantly subject to physical influences from the world around it. In Galenic medicine, the body was made up of (1) 'natural things' (*res naturales*, or elements, humours, faculties and spirits); (2) 'non-natural things' (*res non naturales*, or things external to the body that affect bodily health); and (3) 'things against nature' (*res contra naturam*, or illnesses, their causes and their consequences) (Gentilcore 2016: 14). A healthy body was one in which the four humours (naturals) were perfectly balanced. An unhealthy body, by contrast, was one in which the humours had become discombobulated through exposure to macrocosmic events and situations, for instance food, exercise, fear, unfavourable weather or stagnant and putrid air. Each body was thought to have a particular excess of one humour, which was in turn associated with a particular temperament: an excess of blood made one sanguine (cheerful and easy-going); of phlegm phlegmatic (calm and sluggish); of black bile melancholic (gloomy) and of yellow bile choleric (irritable and quick to anger). Balancing the humours (naturals) involved mastering the six non-naturals (air/environment, food/drink/nutrition, sleep/wakefulness, bodily excretions, movement and emotions) in order to avoid illness (things against nature).

The senses played an important role in this theory, for they formed channels for the macrocosmic phenomena and things to physically enter and impact the body. It was widely thought, for example, that a woman who gave birth to a deformed infant – often understood by contemporaries as 'monsters' – had set eyes upon something ugly or shocking during pregnancy, and the shock from this encounter had caused the physical deformity (Rublack 1996: 94–97). People could likewise fall ill from fear of illness such as plague or from the fear or shock experienced when encountering its manifestations. During the 1664/65 epidemic in Hamburg, the merchant Heusch wrote to his son (who was travelling around Italy) about a woman who had fallen ill from the shock of setting eyes on another woman sick with the plague (Van der Wal 2019: Chapter 18, Letter 9, 27 July 1664). Smell was a particularly important source of good or ill health because what one inhaled was considered material. 'Effluvia', denoting something material that could be perceived via smell, and 'atmosphere' (the air in a space) were key concepts linking smell and health in the eighteenth century (Tullett 2019: 78, 30–32). Effluvia – whether malodourous, sweet-smelling or not detectable to the nose at all – was thought to transmit plague because effluvia carrying contagion ('poison') was believed to be emitted by bodies into the atmosphere, from where it was then breathed in by other bodies (Tullett 2019: 78–80).

Yet plague, for which there was strong Biblical precedent, was also a clear sign of God's wrath. God was thought to 'hold' his 'angered hand over cities and lands' where improper conduct, despair, sin and evil prevailed; ultimately, only His mercy upon the weak human constitution could avert affliction (Anon. 1764: 627–29 [prayer per ordinance to avert contagion, 18 August 1709], translation added). And so, having good health and being a good Christian were inextricably intertwined: bodily order was social order was divine order.

Spaces

These pervasive ideas about the nature of plague, bodies and their interactions had profound implications for the habitation and governance of public spaces in the plague-stricken early modern city. The perceived porosity of bodies and their intimate and unrupturable connection to the environment they inhabited defined and shaped the strategies deployed to manage the existential and spiritual crisis of plague. Certainly, quarantine and isolation played a role, but urban authorities also introduced a number of additional measures that sought not to curb the spread of illness through inhibition of public mobility or the erection of physical barriers, but instead on the maintenance of safe and navigable public spaces.

Like contemporary plague medicine, many municipal reactions to impending plague were prophylactic. One of the first preventative responses undertaken by magistrates when a contagious illness threatened a city was to ensure that public spaces – streets, canals, marketplaces, alleyways and so on – remained free from rubbish and filth that might corrupt the air and propagate contagion. Smell, for the reasons outlined above, was considered particularly problematic. Body collectors and gravediggers, for example, were considered highly susceptible to infection because of the contagious stench emanating from dead bodies (SSA a, 9 November 1710, A3A vol. 42, fol. 363). City authorities fumigated the streets to cleanse the air. Dogs, cats and swine were often slaughtered or removed from the city altogether (SSA a, 25 August 1710, A3A vol. 42, fols 206–09), and householders were routinely ordered to clean their gutters, houses and courtyards and to refrain from disposing of refuse, used bedding or clothes in public spaces (Anon. 1764: Article 8, 822–23 [Contagion Order, 8 September 1713]). The desire for clean and orderly public spaces also extended to people. Hamburg city council, for example, banned households from removing ill persons or 'driving them out into the street' (Anon. 1764: Article 8, 823 [Contagion Order, 8 September 1713], translation added). Social groups thought to transmit infection, such as beggars and Jewish persons, were also routinely kept out of cities (SSA a, 7 December 1710, A3A vol. 42, fols 413–14).

The separation of the healthy from the sick occurred on various fronts, but all measures were designed to ensure that public spaces remained the preserve of the healthy and that public life could continue – as much as possible – in safe environments. The isolation of infected houses and their inhabitants from the outside world for around 40 days was commonplace in cases of feverish, contagious disease. Residents of means were permitted to isolate and quarantine in their households in the countryside. Meanwhile, plague hospitals and pesthouses – often situated outside of the city – were largely the preserve of the poor and destitute, who were unable to provide for themselves in domestic isolation. The movement of healthy persons from households visited by plague was greatly restricted but not always forbidden outright. Healthy householders in Amsterdam, for example, were instructed to take the shortest route through the town to reach the town gates if they fancied a walk (Ancher 1900: 151–53). By contrast, during Hamburg's 1664/65 epidemic, they were banned from wandering streets, markets and 'open spaces or in the churches or other gatherings of healthy people' (Anon. 1763: 215–16 [Instruction on feverish contagious illness, 17 July 1664], translation added).

Preserving the visual integrity of public spaces was also necessary during plague outbreaks, so city authorities introduced further regulations to render plague-afflicted houses and persons readily legible and visible to the urban population. In both Stockholm and Amsterdam, white crosses marked afflicted houses whose inhabitants carried white canes (men) or white handkerchiefs (women) when out in public (Lingelbach 1656; Van der Molen 2020; Stadsarchief Amsterdam 2020; SSA b, vol. F25:14, 1710). In Stockholm, carriages carrying the dead rang bells to keep the people on the streets away (SSA a, 14 October 1710, A3A vol. 42, fols 199–300). Certainly, these signifiers assisted the authorities in calling attention to and keeping track of the diseased, but their purpose was not to instil terror within the beholder (although they may have sometimes had that effect). On the contrary, these markers functioned first and foremost as warning mechanisms for the healthy, allowing them to move through urban thoroughfares whilst steering clear of diseased persons and spaces. In theory, at least, signposting plague during an epidemic made public spaces more predictable, more orderly and more knowable, important benefits during an era in which fear and shock from physical encounters were themselves thought to induce illness.

Sociability

These miasmic understandings of disease and resulting spatial interventions had especially profound implications for intoxicating spaces: inns, taverns, alehouses, coffeehouses and other urban environments specifically designed for physical co-presence and sociability. As the English physician Gideon Harvey (*c*.1636–*c*.1702) put it in 1665, because of 'promiscuous convers[ing] with all sorts of people [...] the contagion oft lights in taverns, ale-houses, &c' (Harvey 1665: 12). Whilst, unlike during the COVID-19 lockdowns, these establishments were never subjected to wholesale closure, they were targeted by emergency legislation across the continent. The 1665 London plague orders were especially explicit on the risks posed by public drinking spaces as vectors of contagion; they described 'disorderly tipling in taverns, alehouses, coffee-houses and cellars' as the 'greatest occasion of dispersing the Plague', and imposed a 9 p.m. curfew (Anon. 1665: sig. B4r). Likewise, a royal proclamation the following year also enjoined that 'no more alehouses be licensed than are absolutely necessary in each city or place' (as part of a wider effort to curb '[p]ublique meetings and concourses of people'), whereas during the 1636 London outbreak, the Royal College of Physicians advised that at infected drinking places 'the signes shall be taken downe for the time of the restraint, and some crosse, or other mark set upon the place thereof to be a token of the sickenesse' (Royal College of Physicians 1636: sig. F3v).

As the language of the 1665 order makes clear – 'the common sin of this time' – the risks posed by intoxicating spaces in times of plague were not purely spatial or physical. Rather, within the providential frameworks described above, by inciting 'swinish drunkenness and gluttony' and related varieties of sinful behaviour, especially on the part of the lower orders, they risked provoking divine retribution in the form of pestilence (Mead 1665: 24). This causal relationship was a frequent refrain in pamphlets published by religious authors during outbreaks. During the 1636 London plague, for example, Puritan medical writer Francis Herring (d.1628) argued that

> concourse of people to stage-playes, wakes or feasts, and May-pole dauncings, are to be prohibited by publique authoritie, whereby as God is dishonored, the bodies of men and women by surfetting, drunkenness, and other riots and excesses, disposed to infection, and the contagion dangerously scattered both in citie and countrie.
> (Herring 1636: sig. A4v)

Likewise, in 1665, the clergyman Richard Kephale explained how in 'tippling houses' and other intoxicating spaces, 'the infection might spread and disperse, by reason of the sin, as well as the commerce and throng of idle sort of persons' (Kephale 1665: 8).

The extent to which these legislative and discursive interventions influenced how people actually used intoxicating spaces during plague times is difficult to determine. Some commentators advised people to avoid them; during the 1625 London outbreak, Stephen Bradwell urged his readers to 'take heed into what houses you enter to drink with your friend: lest instead of a health, you drinke your death. Let every man drinke in his own cup, and let none trust the breath of his brother' (Bradwell 1625: 25). The evidence of ego documents also suggests that intoxicating spaces might indeed have been avoided by the risk-averse. In February 1666, for example, the epidemiologically cautious Samuel Pepys (1633–1703) reported his first visit to a coffeehouse since the outbreak began in the summer of the previous year; however, he expressed surprise that it was 'very full, and company it seems hath been there all the plague time' (Pepys 1666). The evidence from Daniel Defoe's (*c*.1660–1731) celebrated, retrospective account of the 1665 London outbreak, *A Journal of the Plague Year*, is similarly ambiguous. At one point, Defoe observes that

> [t]he gaming tables, publick dancing-rooms, and music-houses which multiply'd [...] were shut up and suppressed; and the jack-puddings, merry-andrews, puppet-shows, rope-dancers, and such like doings [...] shut up their shops, finding indeed no trade [...] death was before their eyes, and every body began to think of their graves, not of mirth and diversions.

However, elsewhere in the account, Defoe devotes several pages to the antics of 'a dreadful set of fellows' at the Pie Tavern, whose proprietors, we learn, 'kept their house open, and their trade going on'. This group of undaunted drinkers 'met there every night, behaved with all the revelling and roaring extravagances, as is usual for such people to do at other times'; they sat in 'a room next the street' and, inter alia, directed 'impudent mocks and jeers' at burial carts and mourners. However, here too the 'hand of God' was at work; all of the revellers were 'struck from heaven with the plague, and died in a most deplorable manner' (Defoe 1722a: 35, 62).

Yet the role of sociability in public spaces was contested and ambiguous; decorous, Christian sociability was desirable and even essential for maintaining the good cheer that, within the medical frameworks outlined above, was necessary to fortify body and soul against infection. Anonymous recommendations on how to mitigate plague published by the Hamburg Council in 1712, for example, argued emphatically for the continuation of public life during epidemics. The author argued that his plans would 'resist the arising fear, as the single cinder of the Plague, and therefore all Conversation amongst the healthy, as well as foreign Commercia, Correspondence and Passage may remain free and open' (Anon. [1712] 2012: n.pag. [Vorrede], translation added). Although he argued against commonplace plague measures such as lazarettos and the shutting up of the stricken – both designed to extricate the sick from public space – the author's reasoning was underpinned by a desire to preserve business as usual and normal public interaction for the healthy. Fear of the plague, he maintained, led the poor to avoid seeking assistance, causing them to drop dead on the street which, in turn, led to a fearful spectacle of plague that frightened the population and drove those of means to flee the city, turning it into a wasteland (Anon. [1712] 2012: n.pag. Chapter 1, § 5). Following his advice, the author argued that

> [p]eople on the street and in Conversation will not face each other with horror, because they know that all those going about the street, are healthy, and people will not drop dead in the street so readily, which would otherwise happen, when the servants and poor people, due to fear of being cast out of the hospital, feel the evil in them, but still remain silent.
> (Anon. [1712] 2012: n.pag. Chap. 2, § 5, IV [2], translation added)

Performances of collective reverence were also encouraged and even expanded in European cities, for group piety was one of the key strategies pursued by both governments and communities in preparing for a contagion. Several pre-epidemic ordinances relate to prayer and church attendance, collective strategies designed to appease God, who would then (hopefully) spare the cities. Dedicated plague prayers were read in churches to both avert and curb the spread of the disease, in conjunction with good dietetic and social comportment. In 1709, the Hamburg council mandated a prayer to be read from the pulpit following regular church services to avert contagion raging to the east and in the Baltic region: 'Spread your wing of mercy over us, so this terror does not near our huts, rather that we may praise your name through pure healthful air, good healthful victuals and drink, blessed medicine and other good situation' (Anon. 1764: 627–29 [Prayer per ordinance to avert the Contagion, 18 August 1709], translation added). The healthy were expected to fulfil the duty of public religious congregation and they did so in large numbers. At no point was there any notion of restricting religious gatherings. In fact, every accommodation was undertaken to augment participation and, at the height of the Hamburg epidemic in 1713, the city council doubled services and confession because the churches were overfilled (Anon. 1764: 812–13 [Announcement of changes to catechism, 7 August 1713]).

Intoxicants

In terms of the unifying logic behind all these plague measures, most were aimed at taming public spaces and rendering them safe. Key to this enterprise were efforts to allay fear, because, as we have seen, a happy and strong body/soul was considered a prerequisite for health and devotion to God. This had major implications for intoxicants (both old and new), which played a central role in official and unofficial medical regimens. They were widely understood to prevent or ameliorate infection by countering noxious air, strengthening the body's key organs (sites of the so-called vital and animal 'spirits'), and, if the individual was infected, by providing antidotes to the poison of plague in the form of powerful counter-toxins. Perhaps most importantly, they possessed analgesic and psychological properties that promised both freedom from physical pain and – maybe more significantly – a degree of relief from the anxiety and emotional torment (or as early modern people would understand it, 'melancholy') induced by pandemic with no cure, which, as we have seen, rendered bodies and minds more vulnerable to infection.

Traditional intoxicants in the form of alcohols – beer, wine and spirits – loomed large in plague repertoires. In Defoe's 1722 treatise *Due Preparations for the Plague* (the lesser-known sister publication to his *Journal of the Plague Year*, published in the same year), he describes 'all manner of provisions' assembled by a prudent London grocer who modelled best practice by voluntarily quarantining himself and his family down for the duration of the 1665 outbreak. His lockdown essentials included

> a reasonable quantity of Wine, Cordial Waters, and Brandy, not for Mirth or plentiful Drinking, but for necessary Supplies, the Physician so having advised, every one that can afford it, to drink moderately; so as not to suffer their Spirits to sink or be dejected as on such melancholy Occasions they might be suppos'd to do.
>
> (Defoe 1722b: 66–68)

Likewise, the natural philosopher Robert Boyle (1627–91) reported the activities of a 'pious and learned schoolmaster' during the same visitation; he visited 1000 infected or dying individuals without injury, his only antidote being the protection of God, a 'constant fearlessness', and 'a spoonful of brandy five or six times a day' (Boyle 1691: 11–13). Perhaps the best single statement on the protective qualities of alcohols when moderately consumed was provided by William Simpson in his 1665 plague treatise *Zenexton anti-pestilentiale*: 'To drink Wine moderately, to make the heart merry, as Solomon saith [...] enlivens the Spirits, and puts the Vitals upon action, so as to stand Centinel against all other bad impressions from malignant Contagions' (Simpson 1665: 8).

The new intoxicants that entered Europe in increasing quantities from the early decades of the seventeenth century also found their way into medical regimens. In plague tractates published in Hamburg, the most common new intoxicants were sugar and tobacco, two substances which, by 1700, were already broadly consumed (Mintz 1992: 115–26). Although a main ingredient in medicinal syrups, sweet substances were considered largely detrimental in plague therapy and used only sparingly (Anon. *c*.1633: n.pag., 25 of digitalization). Sugar, however, was often found in prophylactic preparations. Bökel wrote about 'little sugar cakes' that were prepared by apothecaries and were to be taken 'one or two cakes, sober in the morning, for the evil air, when one wants to go abroad, or to tend the sick' (Bökel 1597: 61v–62v, translation added). Even then, he recognized their addictive potential and advised caution (Bökel 1597: 62v). And yet these plague-evading 'morsels' endured in the prophylactic arsenal and were still touted 100 years later in plague tractates from Hamburg and elsewhere (Kirchoff 1714a).

As with sugar, physicians across Europe recommended tobacco in its various forms as a plague preventative, both for its fumigating properties – a bodily equivalent of the practice of setting bonfires on street corners to sweeten foul urban air – and for its perceived diuretic, drying and purgative effects. As one German commentator put it, 'common smoking tobacco, used in moderation, in both infected areas as in whole armies […] has proven highly effective, and in which many plague epidemics the *Medici* have also preserved and protected themselves' (Kirchoff 1714b: 53, translation added). Keeping dietetic custom – including tobacco consumption – was paramount for robust health: 'Whoever is accustomed to smoking tobacco, would do no harm, if he continues during these times, or even subjects himself more frequently to it' was the medical counsel from the Austrian epidemic (Kirchoff 1714b: 30, translation added; Shapin 2019). Chewing tobacco was also considered a useful prophylactic because it was thought to prevent saliva containing plague poison from being swallowed. People who had to venture amongst the sick were supposed to hold tobacco (as well as other substances such as lovage or lemon rind) in their mouths whilst visiting and tending the ill and then 'dutifully spit it out' afterwards (Kirchoff 1714c: 75, translation added). As with its smoked variety, chewing tobacco could also settle plague-rattled nerves; after seeing several houses in Drury Lane daubed with red crosses early in the 1665 London outbreak, for example, Samuel Pepys was 'put […] into an ill conception of myself and my smell, so that I was forced to buy some roll-tobacco to smell to and chaw, which took away the apprehension' (Pepys 1665).

Although coffee and tea were still used medicinally in the early eighteenth century, in medical texts published in or around the Hamburg epidemic of 1712/13 they functioned more as a supportive dietetic substance. Physicians and other medical writers advised the population to take prophylactics together with tea or coffee (including so-called surrogates or herbal teas) in the morning. As with tobacco, custom – an essential principle of early modern dietetics – was key here: in the morning before going out, one writer advised, 'one can help oneself to chocolate, tea and coffee according to habit' (Kirchoff 1714c: 80; Shapin 2019).

In plague times, then, new intoxicants were more prophylactic than curative. Sugar, tobacco, coffee and tea were part of the dietetic armour that made it possible for bodies to enter public spaces, in which they might encounter a terrible and health-threatening theatre of plague. They did this by fortifying the body, keeping its humours in balance or by removing the dangerous poison. Already a part of everyday habits and diets, including in convivial and pleasurable contexts, these new intoxicants possibly also provided security and comfort in uncertain and bleak times.

Conclusions

Just as COVID-19 made twenty-first century cityscapes places of danger – pathogen-laden assault courses to be negotiated with surgical masks and two-metre exclusion zones – so for the residents of seventeenth-century cities the world beyond the front door became treacherous in plague time. The miasma theory of disease prevalent throughout the period associated infection with 'odious scents', which when inhaled overwhelmed the vital spirits and unbalanced the humours. Moreover, although there was no understanding of the biological mechanisms of transmission – specifically, the rat-borne *yersinia pestis* bacterium that we now know to have been the causative agent of plague – medical writers were fully aware of the possibility of human-to-human contagion via the 'poisonous atmospheres' or 'fatal breath' of the infected ('walking destroyers' in Defoe's striking coinage). On the basis of these understandings, and in the absence of effective cures or vaccines that could protect their citizens, urban authorities implemented a wide range of fundamentally spatial containment measures designed to stop the invisible enemy in its tracks and to render public space safe, legible and navigable for the healthy. This had particular implications for social spaces, yet at the same time, social contact was both a physical and spiritual necessity; sociability had to be accommodated into epidemic life as a matter of moral and health-political necessity. Public spaces were crucial for life-affirming sociability and maintaining good cheer, although not all social spaces were deemed salubrious. Medicines (amongst them intoxicants), diet, prayer and good cheer all served to preserve individual health and the vitality of public life in shared spaces.

ACKNOWLEDGEMENTS

This chapter is based on research undertaken for the research project Intoxicating Spaces: The Impact of New Intoxicants on Urban Spaces in Europe, 1600–1850, funded by HERA as part of its fourth joint research programme Public Spaces: Culture and Integration in Europe (2019–22). The authors would like to thank their project colleagues Karin Sennefelt, Stephen Snelders and Phil Withington for their research on Stockholm, Amsterdam and London that has informed this article.

NOTE

1. Mortality rate for 1713 only. Total mortality in the city was 10,956 in 1713, of which Gernet subtracted 'normal mortality', arriving at between 7000 and 8000 plague dead for a population of around 75,000.

REFERENCES

Anon. (1665), *Orders Conceived and Published by the Lord Major and Aldermen of the City of London, Concerning the Infection of the Plague*, London: James Flesher.

Anon. (1763), *Sammlung der von E. Hochedlen Rathe der Stadt Hamburg sowol zur Handhabung der Gesetze und Verfassungen als bey besondern Eräugnissen in Bürger- und Kirchlichen, auch Cammer-Handlungs- und übrigen Policey-Angelegenheiten und Geschäften vom Anfange des 17. Jahrhunderts bis auf die itzige Zeit ausgegangenen allgemeinen Mandate, bestimmten Befehle und Bescheide, auch beliebten Aufträge und verkündigten Anordnungen; Theil 1 ... welcher die Verfügungen im siebzehnten Jahrhundert in sich fasset*, vol. 1, Hamburg: Piscator.

Anon. (1764), *Sammlung der von E. Hochedlen Rathe der Stadt Hamburg sowol zur Handhabung der Gesetze und Verfassungen als bey besondern Eräugnissen in Bürger- und Kirchlichen, auch Cammer-Handlungs- und übrigen Policey-Angelegenheiten und Geschäften vom Anfange des 17. Jahrhunderts bis auf die itzige Zeit ausgegangenen allgemeinen Mandate, bestimmten Befehle und Bescheide, auch beliebten Aufträge und verkündigten Anordnungen; Theil 2 ... welcher die Verfügungen von 1701 bis 1730 in sich fasset*, vol. 2, Hamburg: Piscator.

Anon. ([c.1633] 2008), *Anmerckungen über D. Johannis Bökelii, Weyland Physici der Stadt Hamburg Pest-Ordnung*, [n.pag.] Göttingen: Göttinger Digitalisierungszentrum, http://resolver.sub.uni-goettingen.de/purl?PPN584686099. Accessed 29 January 2023.

Anon. ([1712] 2012), *Vorschlag, Eines unfehlbahren und Handgreifflich Richtigen Mittels, Der befürchteten und einreissenden Contagion Dergestalt zu begegnen, Daß in jeder Stadt und Dörffern, ohne beschwerliche Kosten, zum wenigsten zwey Drittheil der Häuser von der Infection befreyet bleiben, Die Gesunden und Krancken ihre vollkommene Versorgung erhalten, Der anfallenden Furcht, als den eintzigen Zunder der Pest, Widerstand geschehen, Und demnach Alle Conversation unter denen Gesunden, imgleichen auswärtige Commercia, Correspondenz und Passage frey und offen bleiben könne*, Hamburg: Thomas von Wierings Erben, Göttingen: Niedersächsische Staats- und Universitätsbibliothek.

Ancher, Aloysius Brouwer (1900), 'De pest en hare bestrijding in vroeger eeuwen', W. G. C. Byvanck, J. N. van Hall, A. G. van Hamel, A. W. Hubrecht, G. Kalff, W. L. P. A. Molengraaff and R. P. J. Tutein Nolthenius (eds), in *De Gids*, vol. 64, Amsterdam: P.N. van Kampen and Zoon, pp. 148–78, digitale bibliotheek voor de Nederlandse letteren, https://www.dbnl.org/tekst/_gid001190001_01/_gid001190001_01_0006.php?q=brouwer#hl1. Accessed 29 January 2023.

Barbette, Paul (1687), *Thesaurus Chirgurgiae: The Chirurgical and Anatomical Works of Paul Barbette Composed According to the Doctrine of the Circulation of the Blood, and Other New Inventions of the Moderns: Together with a Treatise of the Plague, Illustrated with Observations / Translated Out Of Low-Dutch Into English ...; To Which Is Added The Surgeon's Chest, Furnished Both with Instruments And Medicines ... And to Make It More Compleat, Is Adjoyned a Treatise of Diseases That for the Most Part Attend Camps and Fleets; Written in High-Dutch by Raymundus Minderius*, 4th ed., London: Henry Rodes.

Benedictow, Ole Jørgen (1987), 'Morbidity in historical plague epidemics', *Population Studies*, 41:3, pp. 401–31.

Bökel, Johannes (1597), *Pestordnung der Stadt Hamburg. D. Iohannis Bökelij Physici daselbst*, Hamburg: Jacob Lucius der Jüngere.

Boyens, Kathrin (2004), 'Die Krise in der Krise. Die Maßnahmen Hamburgs während der letzten Pest 1712–1714', in O. Ulbricht (ed.), *Die leidige Seuche. Pest-Fälle in der Frühen Neuzeit*, Cologne: Böhlau Verlag, pp. 295–325.

Boyle, Robert (1691), *Experimenta and Observationes Physicae*, London: John Taylor & John Wyat.

Bradwell, Stephen (1625), *A Watch-Man for the Pest*, London: George Vincent.

Champion, Justin (1995), *London's Dreaded Visitation: The Social Geography of the Great Plague of London, 1665*, Edinburgh: University of Edinburgh.

Cohn, Samuel and Alfani, Guido (2007), 'Households and plague in early modern Italy', *The Journal of Interdisciplinary History*, 38:2, pp. 177–205.

Cruikshank, George (1833), *A Cart for Transporting the Dead in London During the Great Plague*, London: Wellcome Collection, 6922i, https://wellcomecollection.org/works/hjbr8cxs. Accessed 29 January 2023.

Defoe, Daniel (1722a), *A Journal of the Plague Year*, London: E. Nuttm J. Roberts, A. Dodd, & J. Graves.

Defoe, Daniel (1722b), *Due Preparations for the Plague, as well for Soul as Body*, London: E. Matthews & J. Batley.

Dinges, Martin (1995), 'Pest und Staat: Von der Institutionsgeschichte zur sozialen Konstruktion?' in M. Dinges and T. Schlich (eds), *Neue Wege in der Seuchengeschichte*, Stuttgart: Steiner Verlag, pp. 71–104.

Dinges, Martin and Schlich, Thomas (eds) (1995), *Neue Wege in der Seuchengeschichte*, Stuttgart: Steiner Verlag.

Evans, Hilary and Evans, Mary (1978), *The Man Who Drew the Drunkard's Daughter: The Life and Art of George Cruikshank, 1792–1878*, London: Frederick Muller Limited.

Gentilcore, David (2016), *Food and Health in Early Modern Europe: Diet, Medicine and Society, 1450–1800*, London: Bloomsbury Academic.

Gernet, Hermann G. ([1869]), *Mittheilungen aus der älteren Medicinalgeschichte Hamburg's. Kulturhistorische Skizze auf urkundlichem und geschichtlichem Grunde*, Hamburg: [Mauke] Staats- und Universitätsbibliothek Hamburg, Hamburger Kulturgut Digital, https://resolver.sub.uni-hamburg.de/kitodo/PPN623454815. Accessed 29 February 2023.

Harvey, Gideon (1665), *A Discourse of the Plague Containing the Nature, Causes, Signs, and Presages of the Pestilence in General, Together with the State of the Present Contagion*, London: Nathan Brooke.

Herring, Francis (1636), *Certaine Rules, Directions, or Advertisements for This Time of Pestilentiall Contagion*, London: Thomas Paine.

Hodges, Nathaniel (1720), *Loimologia: Or, an Historical Account of the Plague in London in 1665*, London: E. Bell & J. Osborn.

Jones, Colin (1996), 'Plague and its metaphors in early modern France', *Representations*, 53: Winter, pp. 97–127.

Kephale, Richard (1665), *Medela Pestilentiae Wherein is Contained Several Theological Queries Concerning the Plague, with Approved Antidotes, Signes and Symptoms*, London: Samuel Speed.

Kemp, William (1665), *A Brief Treatise of the Nature, Causes, Signes, Preservation from, and Cure of the Pestilence Collected by W. Kemp*, London: D. Kemp.

Kirchoff, Gottfried (1714a), *Vier Tractätlein von der ansteckenden Seuche, welche Anno 1713. In das Ertz-Hertzogthum Nieder-Oesterreich eingeschlichen. Der Werthen Stadt Hamburg und allen Nieder-Sachsen zu Liebe und Dienst; Nebst einer Vorrede Von einer schädlichen Pest-Medicin*, Hamburg: Liebezeit.

Kirchoff, Gottfried (1714b), 'Ansteckender Seuche, Welche dieses 1713. Jahr In das Ertz-Hertzogthum Nieder-Oesterreich eingeschlichen, Gründliche und ausführliche Nachricht, sonderbar aus das Land Sammt benöthigten Hülffs-Rettungs- und Verwahrungs-Mitteln. Aus dem Nieder-Oestereichischen Gesundheits-Rath', in G. Kirchoff, *Vier Tractätlein von der ansteckenden Seuche*, Hamburg: Liebezeit, p. 30.

Kirchoff, Gottfried (1714c), 'Gantz Kurtzer und Deutlicher Aufsatz, Wie Sich der gemeine Mann und Arme wider die Gegenwärtige in N. Oe. An etlichen Orten, gifftig= und sehr ansteckende Seuche, Wo sonst kein Rath, noch Artzt vorhanden, selbst schützen und heilen kann. Von Ein=auftichtigem Freund derer Armen entworffen', in G. Kirchoff (ed.), *Vier Tractätlein von der ansteckenden Seuche*, Hamburg: Liebezeit, p. 106.

Kümin, Beat and Usborne, Cornelie (2013), 'At home and in the workplace: A historical introduction to the "spatial turn"', *History and Theory*, 52:3, pp. 305–18.

Lingelbach, Johannes (1656), *De Dam, gezien naar het Noorden, met het Stadhuis in aanbouw*, SA 3044, Amsterdam: Amsterdam Museum, http://hdl.handle.net/11259/collection.38042. Accessed 29 January 2023.

Mead, Matthew (1665), *Solomon's Prescription for the Removal of the Pestilence, Or, The Discovery of the Plague of Our Hearts, in Order to the Healing of That in Our Flesh*, London: Matthew Mead.

Mignon, Abraham (c.1670), *Still Life with Rotting Fruit and Nuts on a Stone Ledge*, Cambridge: The Fitzwilliam Museum, https://data.fitzmuseum.cam.ac.uk/id/object/3027. Accessed 29 January 2023.

Mintz, Sydney W. (1992), *Die süße Macht. Kulturgeschichte des Zuckers*, Frankfurt Main: Campus-Verlag.

Newman, Kira L. S. (2012), 'Shutt up: Bubonic plague and quarantine in early modern England', *Journal of Social History*, 45:3, pp. 809–34.

Ornell, Felipe, Moura, Helena Ferreira, Scherer, Juliana Nichterwitz, Pechansky, Flavio, Kessler, Felix Henrique Paim and von Diemen, Lisia (2020), 'The COVID-19 pandemic and its impact on substance use: Implications for prevention and treatment', *Psychiatry Research*, 289:113096, n.pag., https://doi.org/10.1016/j.psychres.2020.113096.

Pepys, Samuel (1665), 'Wednesday 7 June 1665', *The Diary of Samuel Pepys*, https://www.pepysdiary.com/diary/1665/06/07/. Accessed 19 March 2023.

Pepys, Samuel (1666), 'Friday 16 February 1665/66', *The Diary of Samuel Pepys*, https://www.pepysdiary.com/diary/1666/02/16/. Accessed 19 March 2023.

Quincy, John (1721), *An Essay on the Different Causes of Pestilential Diseases, and How They Became Contagious*, London: E. Bell & J. Osborn.

Royal College of Physicians (1636), *Certain Necessary Directions, as Well for the Cure of the Plague as for Preventing the Infection*, London: John Bill & Christopher Barker.

Rublack, Ulinka (1996), 'Pregnancy, childbirth and the female body in early modern Germany', *Past & Present*, 150: February, pp. 84–110.

Simpson, William (1665), *Zenexton Anti-pestilentiale*, London: George Sawbridge.

Shapin, Simon (2019), 'Why was "custom a second nature" in early modern medicine?' *Bulletin of the History of Medicine*, 93:1, pp. 1–26.

Slack, Paul (1985), *The Impact of Plague in Tudor and Stuart England*, London: Routledge.

Slack, Paul (1988), 'Responses to plague in early modern Europe: The implications of public health', *Social Research*, 55:3, pp. 433–53.

Stadsarchief Amsterdam (2020), 'Epidemie-bestrijding in de zeventiende eeuw', *Nieuws*, 14 April, https://www.amsterdam.nl/stadsarchief/nieuws/epidemie/. Accessed 29 January 2023.

Stockholm City Archive (SSA): (a) Stockholms magistrat och rådhusrätt, Civilprotokoll, huvudserie, 25 August 1710, A3A vol. 42, fols 206–9; 14 October 1710, A3A vol. 42, fols 299–300; 9 November 1710, A3A vol. 42, fol. 363; 4 November 1710, A3A vol. 42, fol. 350; 7 December 1710, A3A vol. 42, fols 413–14. (b) Stockholms magistrat och rådhusrätt, Övriga ämnesordnade handlingar, vol. F25:14, 1710.

Tullett, William (2019), *Smell in Eighteenth-Century England: A Social Sense*, Oxford: Oxford University Press.

UNICEF Data Hub (2023), 'COVID-19 and children', https://data.unicef.org/covid-19-and-children/. Accessed 29 January 2023.

University of Glasgow Library (n.d.), 'Dancing with Death. The origins and development of the Dance of Death motif and its representation in graphic art: the Gemmell Collection at the University of Glasgow Library', Special Collections, https://www.gla.ac.uk/myglasgow/library/files/special/exhibns/death/deathhome.html. Accessed 29 January 2023.

Van der Molen, Tom (2020), 'De Dam tijdens een epidemie. Onzichtbaar gevaar in 1656', Blog Amsterdam Museum, 14 April, https://hart.amsterdam/nl/page/1053442/de-dam-tijdens-een-epidemie. Accessed 29 January 2023.

Van der Wal, Marijke (2019), *Koopmanszoon Michiel Heusch op Italiëreis: Brieven van het thuisfront (1664–1665)*, Hilversum: Verloren.

COVID-19: TEXTS AND DISCOURSE

8

Coronavirus in Times of the Late Internet: Compulsive Visualization and a Data-Hungry Society

Agnieszka Jelewska

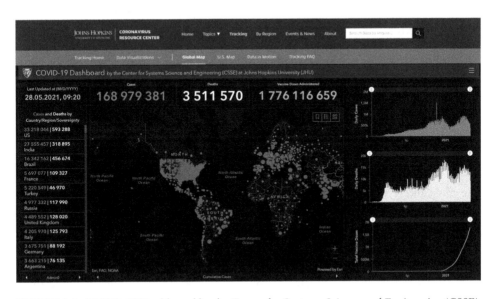

FIGURE 8.1: COVID-19 Dashboard by the Center for Systems Science and Engineering (CSSE) at Johns Hopkins University, screenshot from 28 May 2021.

In today's world, the methods of managing crises, plagues and diseases have a techno-biological dimension – the mechanisms of constructing and distributing information about these phenomena are just as important as the spread of the virus (Parikka 2007). With the COVID-19 pandemic,[1] we can observe important feedback processes at work in aspects of life and specific sciences – on the one hand, health, life and corporeality, on the other, medical technology and communication technologies. This is not a state of exception since, as Michel Foucault wrote, a pandemic is always an exceptional state that brings biopolitics and anatomo-politics closer together, dangerously abolishing the boundaries between them (Foucault 2008), and because 'restrictions are placed on certain transmissions (circulating bodies); periodic biomedical interventions are normalized and accepted in order to preserve life' (Sundaram 2021: n. pag.). What we have observed from the very inception of this pandemic, however, is that the technologies themselves have very quickly become medicalized and bodies and lives technologized. Since the arrival of COVID-19, our interaction with digital technology has increased to unprecedented levels (Fuchs 2021), linking together various spheres of human functioning in a state of emergency – from healthcare, through the economic crisis and the disclosure of political radicalism, to a strong hybridization of the private and digital spheres in the situation of lockdown (Coeckelbergh 2020). The circumstances surrounding this feedback can be traced by analysing the role of digital technologies (applications, websites, maps, interactive graphics and visualizations), which – as modes of the rapid flow of information and data dissemination, not only by mainstream media but also through various internet platforms – have revealed new levels of knowledge production with the use of technologies, not only concerning the pandemic itself but also its effects and projected consequences for the future functioning of societies (Lee et al. 2021). This double entanglement made important contributions to a new understanding of the agency of digital technological systems, not so much in terms of solving the problem of the pandemic, because vaccines were created in closed laboratories in a race between pharmacological companies, but rather in its modelling, prediction and visualization and in communicating what was allowed or not allowed, how the virus would spread, who was responsible for it, etc.

At the forefront of producing knowledge about the pandemic and predicting the most likely ways that the virus would evolve were not only the virological experts who gave numerous media interviews and whose statements, quoted and commented on in very different ways, flooded social networks (Anderson 2022), but also computer scientists, mathematicians and AI modellers, who predicted the next waves of infection, and experts responsible for visualizing data on the spread of the virus, the number of infected people and deaths. As Sara Callaghan described, 'Covid 19 is a data science issue' (Callaghan 2020). Due to the global dimension of the pandemic, expert knowledge about the disease and its effects was automated very rapidly. This was responsible for global data dissemination, in the multidimensional form of maps, dashboards, diagrams and graphics. So, the pandemic has generated – and also sanctioned – the existence of human-inhuman experts. The knowledge designed by scientists was closely combined with extensive AI algorithmic systems and ways of visualizing data. This entanglement of new modes of knowledge production can be analysed through the hundreds of methods of data visualization which we were able to observe day after day during the pandemic. These visualizations were produced to satisfy the hunger for information that arose as a result of the lack of transparent forms of communication between expert knowledge and societies.

The aim of this text is to identify the epistemic gap which emerged between visualizations based on pandemic data and its social perception and understanding as a problematic sphere for the formation of knowledge in a data-driven and data-hungry society. This gap is epistemological in nature and relates not only to the pandemic (although this is what revealed the deficiency) but also to the broader problem we face today: the crisis of expert knowledge in relation to accelerated forms of technological production, reproduction and replication.

The starting point for the considerations in this chapter is the COVID-19 Dashboard created by the Center of System Science and Engineering at Johns Hopkins University (see Figure 8.1), which, from the very first days of the pandemic, due to its visualizations of the spread of the virus, became an icon of knowledge production through algorithmic analyses of big data. Everyone is no doubt familiar with the red dots of varying sizes that, since the arrival of COVID-19, have grown inside the black outlines of schematic continents. The project, initiated by Ensheng Dong, a doctoral student from Johns Hopkins University, was an iconic dashboard visualization, based on the Geographic Information System, that allowed the spread of the pandemic to be mapped and tracked in terms of the number of infected people and deaths (Dong et al. 2020). In the first period of the pandemic, it served as the main tool for many countries to analyse and disseminate knowledge about virus behaviour and its consequences on human lives. However, this visualization strategy was not simply a form of showing the course of the pandemic: it became a kind of infrastructure for the production of knowledge about morbidity and mortality, and it generated specific political, intra-state and global responses (e.g. through the WHO) in the form of new restrictions, prevention measures and data collection methods. This dashboard also added a certain aesthetic to the public's perception of the pandemic in its first weeks. 'Along with lists of total counts and histograms, a bubble map composed of circles of different radii allows a visual inspection of how serious the pandemic is around the world' (Comba 2020: 81). It was this manner of visualization, which was based on two colour palettes of red and black and the dynamics of incremental red spheres, that incorporated, throughout the infrastructure it produced, the effects and emotions of the viewer.

The colour scheme and the way the data were visualized became a way to manage levels of anxiety in specific areas of the Earth. 'We're constantly adjusting the dots', said Dong (Milner 2020: 57), referring to the early days of this dashboard.

> We added a few other maps besides the cumulative and confirmed cases, such as active cases, to clearly communicate the data we were collecting and sharing. If more people in your country are recovering, you refer to that map. The dots are smaller, and you feel better.
> (Milner 2020: 57)

This way of approaching the issue turned the virus into an onto-technological object: it not only had a physical impact on human life but also replicated itself in this visualization, creating an image of a dark planet flooded with red balls of different sizes. The style adopted in the dashboard, taken straight from apocalyptic graphics, certainly did not facilitate a broader understanding of the pandemic processes that we had to face and which we could not really understand in the absence of certain knowledge from experts, virologists, doctors, researchers and vaccine developers. Before we even had a clear idea of what was really going on, the pandemic had been visually reduced to an interactive dashboard with daily versions transmitted and commented on in mainstream media and on social media platforms. This obscured the real problems that were emerging due to the increasing number of cases in certain places and communities in favour of a simplified, visually paralysing global picture of the pandemic. The initial lack of access to detailed data and the absence of extended applications that explained the ways in which data were captured within the Johns Hopkins University dashboard (which was later supplemented with additional functions) did not allow users to penetrate the layers of visualization. In a sense, recipients remained on the surface of the interactive image. Confused by the situation, which experts were unable to explain precisely, in the absence of vaccines, which were supposed to be the only remedy, users looked at the image of the impending end of the world, which, according to the visuality of the Johns Hopkins University dashboard, was actually already happening. These vibrantly coloured and simplified visualizations also somehow caused users to lose their sense of the reality of disease and death, since these were viewed through a dynamic image of dots. After all, the dots did not represent specific victims of the pandemic. Moreover, the combination of such visuality with the rapid development of surveillance policies in the early stages of the pandemic (deep lockdown in the first months and subsequent changes in national strategies) as well as the lack of reliable information and erratic changes in its interpretation (e.g. WHO's confusing guidance on masks at the very beginning of the COVID-19 pandemic [Chan et al. 2020]) generated situations in which the virus was treated as an onto-technological product – touching life but technologically managed, disclosed and transmitted. Subsequent rapid responses to this visuality included interactive dashboards and other additional tools for analysing COVID-19 data that were prepared by teams from the *New York Times* and the *Washington Post*. The former used bright colours with transparent visual textures in white, yellow, orange and light red. The gradation of colours and the translucency of the forms allowed viewers to become accustomed to the map and encouraged extended interaction by means of the available tools. The *New York Times* used chronopleth maps, which, among other things, displayed the time series evolution for each region using linear heat maps, where daily values were mapped as colours and displayed in a row. However, these maps failed to also address the epistemic gap that emerged between knowledge, data and the public understanding and reception of these processes, as a result of which users defined and spun stories about the coronavirus. What is more, the *New York Times* map was at times overloaded and complicated and thus perpetuated essentially stereotypical ways of mapping data in an attractive but also highly globalized format.

Figure 8.1 shows the COVID-19 Dashboard by the Center for Systems Science and Engineering (CSSE) at Johns Hopkins University (screenshot from 28 May 2021).[2] In the case of the data visualizations made by Johns Hopkins University, in addition to these psychosomatic problems, other issues related to the production of knowledge about the pandemic came to light. The cartographer Alan McConchie wrote,

> despite being one of the most reliable sources of COVID data and charts, [it] also had one of the most misinterpreted COVID maps. At times, it felt like everyone on social media who works with maps found themselves at some point explaining to people how they were reading it wrong.
>
> (McConchie 2021b: n.pag.)

A widely discussed problem with the Johns Hopkins map, as McConchie points out, was its inconsistent level of detail. This was due to the fact that the map used data from the various locations from which they were collected while failing to indicate these varied origins in its visualization strategies and without referencing the data to the spatial contexts from which they emerged. A famous example analysed by researchers concerned the red dots on the border of the United States and Canada. In the United States, the modes of data collection referred to larger units, such as counties, so during the peak of each wave of the pandemic, there were a great many small red dots. However, in the case of Canada, the data were aggregated by province, so there was only one dot in the middle of each province. This gave the impression that infections stopped at the United States border, which was not consistent with the reality experienced by border residents in Canada. 'The data on the map is not wrong, but it is very misleading', commented McConchie (2021b).

Imagine if the tables were turned: if Canada's rate were twice the US, but it was still only mapped by province in Canada and by county in the US, you would still see more red on the map in the United States and think things were worse here.

(McConchie 2021a: n.pag.)

Alberto Cairo, author of *How Charts Lie. Getting Smarter about Visual Information*, commenting on Twitter about the misleading visualization of the Johns Hopkins dashboard, suggested that the problem lies in the fact that the map shows data at different levels of aggregation: sometimes there is one circle per country, sometimes, as in the United States, one per county. In addition, the counties are not proportional to size. Part of the reason for this is the different sizes of the area: large and sparsely populated states may look more prominent than small states with a high population density (Cairo 2020).

The example of the Johns Hopkins map is just one of the many types of visualizations that emerged during the pandemic. Nevertheless, it has proved to epitomize rapid data visualization, as it was one of the first to be disseminated in the global media. This project is symptomatic of a broader issue related to the growing modes of data visualization during the pandemic and their public perception and understanding. The rapid development of visualization strategies was dictated by the vast amounts of incoming data generated on a global scale. Consequently, some strategies failed to take into account extreme diversity (in terms of racial, economic and legal factors, the demographic specificity of the area from which the data came and the methods of data collection), some strategies paid insufficient attention to aggregation methodologies and others gave little thought to how the visualizations themselves should be introduced into the social debate. The pandemic provided an extremely blunt illustration of the saying 'data are never raw' (Gitelman 2013); neither are they free from interpretation and explanation at any level – different factors are involved in how data are collected and processed, as well as in the choice of visualization strategy appropriate to them.

Platform pandemic: Misleading data stories on the late internet

During the COVID-19 pandemic, algorithmic precognition played an increasingly important role. Mathematical models that functioned as precognitions in the culture of epidemics began to be treated not as probable scenarios of events, but as strategies for managing knowledge and telling stories about the future of the pandemic and seemed to introduce the concept of 'being with a crisis' into the everyday functioning of citizens. This opened up and accelerated the tendency to speculate using data, which is very characteristic of the 'late internet'. The latter is a concept that refers to the period of 'late capitalism', where a great deal of energy and action goes into speculation and pseudo-transactions rather than producing or creating new goods and services (Michie 2020). The late internet age facilitates speculation using data, and information has become the primary 'commodity'. This situation was powerfully illustrated by the COVID-19 pandemic, which triggered further crises and concerns, expressed in very different ways:

> the pandemic has accelerated all antinomies of the system: unprecedented platform power and collective responses to medical crisis; the crisis of neoliberal austerity and unapparelled monetary intervention by Western regimes; racial violence and global countermovements; the normalization of surveillance technologies with biomedical interventions and constantly shifting boundaries of the 'normal'; the proliferation of hate speech and an extraordinary investment in scientific authority.
>
> (Sundaram 2021: 4–5)

The whole nexus of events, reactions and situations that the pandemic generated should also be seen from a perspective that considers the internet as an infrastructure of late capitalism, i.e. a space for the flow of countless data about the pandemic that was spread, generated, visualized and commented on online. As a virulent disease, COVID-19 was spread through air or sea travel or interpersonal communication in general, but as a techno-biological condition, it also became a product of the late internet. There was thus a rapid process of the platformization of the pandemic, enabling the flow of the most diverse data and ways of visualizing and commenting on it, which not only broadened the scope of scientific knowledge about the pandemic but also provided the basis for misleading data stories to spread in the media and on social media platforms.

One such example was analysed by a research team from the Massachusetts Institute of Technology. The paper *Viral Visualizations: How Coronavirus Skeptics Use Orthodox Data Practices to Promote Unorthodox Science Online* addressed the issue of how opponents of mask mandates used forms of data visualization to question the effectiveness of wearing masks. The team analysed how data visualizations circulated on social media from the beginning of the pandemic and showed that people who distrust scientific discourse often use the same rhetoric and methodology for data visualizations that experts use. However, they use them differently to support their own political and economic agendas. Using a quantitative analysis of how visualizations spread on Twitter and an ethnographic approach to analysing conversations on COVID-19 data on Facebook, the research team demonstrated that pro- and anti-mask groups 'draw drastically different inferences from similar data' (Lee et al. 2021: 1). As part of their research, anti-mask groups were found to practice 'a form of data literacy in spades'. The anti-mask groups revealed themselves as prolific producers and consumers of data visualization, and their diagrams closely resembled those used by researchers. Their approaches to visualization did not indicate a lack of skill with these strategies; in fact, the opposite is true: sophisticated data visualization practices became a means of consolidating and disseminating views that were false. Importantly, however, as a result of the research, the team found that quantitative overviews of the visualizations shared and amplified by anti-masks groups do not in themselves 'help to understand how they invoke data and scientific reasoning to support policies like re-opening schools and businesses' (Lee et al. 2021: 10).

This means that such data visualizations were made without transparent indication of the origin of the data and the methodologies of their aggregation. Thus, we were dealing with a situation in which the very aesthetics of the image or interactive graphics resembled those used by scientific centres. However, this was done without any indication of which data were subject to analysis. This situation proved to be unprecedented. As data visualizations by geographers, cartographers, virologists and others became an extremely important part of knowledge production during the pandemic, they circulated online and created what I call an epistemic gap between a data-hungry society and the visualization interfaces. These visualizations did not have the necessary 'settings' to explain the origins of the data or the process through which they were retrieved and analysed, so this gap resulted in different COVID-sceptic groups using aesthetic images in isolation for the purpose of visualizing their own data and shaping them to suit their own political beliefs. This points to the wider problem that science faces in constructing knowledge by means of data-driven strategies, particularly when data are collected and quickly visualized without the social process being revealed or explained. As the researchers point out in not only *Viral Visualizations*, 'throughout the coronavirus pandemic, researchers have held up the crisis as a "breakthrough moment" for data visualization research'; however, no work has been done to take into account the social understanding of the data and the visualization processes themselves, 'as the discussion around COVID datasets and visualizations are manifestations of deeper political questions about the role of science in public life' (Lee et al. 2021: 3). The gap in question points to the need to develop concepts of interdisciplinary and even transdisciplinary collaborations (involving communities outside the scientific system) to rethink and develop new cultures of data analysis and visualization as co-designers of wider cultures of knowledge. A key part of this shift would include sharing data with other disciplines at an early level of working with data – particularly the more analytical and critical disciplines, such as environmental humanities, critical sociology and media studies, and this process should involve those for whom visualizations are designed.

Data are local and must be situated closer to the people

The problem of the relationship between data and its visualization is not new. During the pandemic, due to the hunger for data on a global and local scale, which was then 'digested' by individuals, countries and global organizations, the processes of rapid visualization of all data underwent considerable development. Therefore, as I mentioned, the problem of a lack of data localization and public understanding of the visualization process proved to be extremely acute, requiring urgent consideration. In his book, *All Data Are Local: Thinking Critically in a Data-Driven Society*, published a year before the pandemic, the designer and data scientist Yanni Alexander Loukissas had already drawn attention to the ongoing discussion about the social and political implications of automated data aggregation. As he highlighted, data that are disconnected from local conditions and contexts are subject to homogenization and algorithmic consolidation. Differences between individual data, which are only perceived from a situated perspective, cease to be taken into account at all. This is because algorithmization is linked to processes of abstraction. This problem was also pointed out by Ed Finn: 'Algorithms enact theoretical ideas in pragmatic instructions, always leaving a gap between the two in the details of implementation' (2017: 2). This results in falsifications and internal conflicts within the dataset. Subjected to automatic visualization, the dataset is thus linked to a homogenizing aesthetics that aims to subjugate the results obtained and subordinate them to a preconceived cognitive framework.

In *'Missing/Unspecified': Demographic Data Visualization During the COVID-19 Pandemic*, Rachel Atherton draws attention to the cognitive deficiencies that were caused by the top-down approach to data visualization that dominated the media and public opinion. She points out that the prevailing mainstream data visualizations, such as those produced by Johns Hopkins University, excluded a great many factors relating to demographics that could be considered relevant for understanding the consequences of the pandemic for specific communities. Using the United States as an example, she makes clear that there was a process of disconnection between reported datasets and data visualizations in public-facing COVID-19 health and science communications. In the case of the United States, most visualizations tended to highlight how different groups, particularly marginalized ones, were affected by COVID-19, but their national focus did not allow users to investigate the virus's impact on their own communities. Broad claims are useful in certain contexts or for national organizations, such as the Center for Disease Control and Prevention, but citizens interested in taking action locally need local data (Atherton 2021: 85). Consequently, 'data reifies existing power structures and inequalities' (Atherton 2021: 80). It is therefore important, writes Atherton, that 'technical and professional communicators take steps in creating or using data visualizations accurately and ethically to describe COVID conditions and impacts' (2021: 80). She, therefore, suggests that we should consider not only what answers are provided by specific data visualizations but also what questions they completely fail to answer.

> If the visualization's answers do not include questions about marginalized communities, we must ask why and consider if and how they can be expanded accordingly. Data is created, not found, so marginalized communities must be considered and included before the data is even collected; otherwise, we might not have inclusive data available to visualize, as in the absence of nearly 80% of the CDC's racial data.
> (Atherton 2021: 86)

One example of an attempt to tackle the issue of the ethics of visualizations and their public understanding is an interdisciplinary project initiated by the Collective for Open Data Distribution-Keralam (CODD-K), an international consortium which brings together dozens of researchers from different disciplines, including physics, mathematics, geography, cognitive science, software programming, genetics, geophysics, sociology and psychiatry. CODD-K created a citizen science-based project for open data that focused on the incidence and development of the pandemic in Kerala, India. The research used a wide variety of publicly available data on the COVID-19 epidemic in specific areas of Kerala, such as government bulletins and information published in the media and various news outlets. In the first stage, open reusable datasets were generated. The project team then visualized these as a dashboard via a front-end web application and within a JavaScript Object Notation (JSON) repository, which serves as the application programming interface for the user interface (Ulahannan et al. 2020: 1913). Data from multiple sources were refined to create a structured live dataset and provide real-time analysis and daily updates of COVID-19 cases in Kerala through a bilingual (English and Malayalam) user-friendly dashboard.[3] The aim was to disseminate data on epidemic trends, places with the highest number of infectious and daily statistics in a way that could be understood by non-specialists and to include bilingual interpretations. Importantly, the data were not aggregated in a way that prevented contextual definition and reuse. The researchers wanted the datasets to be usable, so they placed them in a public repository, following the principles of open data, for future analytical activities and processes of verification and re-description (Ulahannan et al. 2020: 1914). Volunteer citizens were also invited to participate in the project. The data collection process was transparent and the data were not homogeneous; they were collected from different sources and were subjected to open validation procedures:

> The domain experts in the collective defined the data of interest to be collected, established the informatics workflow, and the Web application for data visualization. The

volunteers contributed by sourcing data from various media outlets for enriching the data. Social media channels (Telegram channels and WhatsApp groups) were used for data collection, which was verified independently and curated by data validation team members. [...] The collective defined the data of interest as minimal structured metadata of the COVID-19 infections in Kerala, covering the possible facets of its spatial and temporal nature, excluding the clinical records.

(Ulahannan et al. 2020: 1915)

These data were structured into described sets that were linked together in accordance with specific definitional elements. They were then visualized using a dashboard and, together with the associated source codes, customized and made available as open-source software under the MIT licence. The whole process – from collection through analysis to description, the methodology responsible for creating links between datasets and the visualization strategy – was based on transparency, openness at every stage (including visualizations) and data reusability. This means that it is possible to analyse the visualizations and move to different levels of data definition. Thus, the knowledge we can obtain throughout the analysis is spatially and temporally situated as a heterogeneous multilevel and open structure. The bilingual online dashboard not only presents a variety of data on deaths, illnesses, recoveries, etc., but its creators have also responded to user feedback on an ongoing basis, adding new graphs and visualizations based on recommendations. Importantly, as a consequence of the whole project, there was also 'a manually curated data archive maintained as a GitHub repository for the provenance' (Ulahannan et al. 2020: 1916). In this project, the process of data curation was carried out with the understanding that data are neither raw nor objective, so a specific culture of analysis and visualization needs to be created for them. Data are situated, and open ways of accessing and sharing them are required. The citizen-led collective work that the project accomplished in Kerala specifically addressed the challenges of data curation and thus gained a wider understanding and openness to social interaction.

Data curation and interdisciplinary modes of visualization

In the book referred to above, Loukissas describes ways of working with data based on the concept of 'curation' (from the Latin *cura*, meaning 'care'), encapsulating them in six basic principles:

1. Look at the data setting, not just the data set.
2. Make place a part of the data presentation.
3. Take a comparative approach to data analysis.

4. Challenge normative algorithms using counterdata.
5. Create interfaces that cause friction.
6. Use data to build relationships.

(Loukissas 2019: 4)

The process of curation is not possible without extended ethnographic fieldwork; it is only in this way that digital data can be situated in a local context. 'More experimentally, reading locally can mean imagining how data might be seen in new ways, using speculative yet nevertheless locally imagined modes of visualization' (Loukissas 2019: 8). Situated data produce 'friction' and require new, non-normative and non-homogenizing methods of analysis and visualization. Loukissas considers data and the forms of their visualization as a 'point of contact' or an opportunity 'to get closer, to learn to care about a subject or the people and places beyond data' (2019: 196). As such, data must be analysed in context and as a kind of 'text' or cultural expression that is 'subject to interpretive examination' (2019: 7). He, therefore, extends the very process of data analysis, not only returning it to its local spatio-temporal conditions but also to its cultural determinants. This is a very important aspect of knowledge production gained by data-driven visualization. Moreover, the lack of developed awareness of the diversity of cultural perceptions of visualization very often also leads users from a given culture to misunderstand the visual language employed in representing the data.

A wide-ranging approach to the issue of data visualization, referring not only to the pandemic itself but also to its consequences for specific communities, excluded people, human and non-human subjects, as well as new problems generated by this situation, is provided by a curatorial project initiated by the environmental humanities scholar Sria Chatterjee and carried out in collaboration with Critical Media Lab (Basel, Switzerland), Princeton Center for Digital Humanities (Princeton University), Institute of Experimental Design and Media FHNW Academy of Art and Design (Basel, Switzerland).[4] *Visualizing the Virus* is a constantly-evolving platform for collecting experimental ways of visualizing data on COVID-19; a multicultural digital project that focuses on understanding the pandemic from different perspectives. As the researchers suggest, publicly available visualizations of the pandemic have lacked the support of inter- and transdisciplinary projects that attempt to bridge the distance that has arisen between the humanities, social sciences and natural sciences. Hence, '*Visualizing the Virus* connects insights from different disciplines to create a collective digital space for exactly such a convergence' (Chatterjee 2020: n.pag.). Both the data and the forms of visualization are very different – among the numerous examples, we can find the following: *Cartography of COVID-19* by Dario Rodighiero, Eveline Wandl-Vogt, Elian Carsenat (visualization of the links between scientific articles on COVID-19 from the COVID-19 Open Research Dataset in the form of a semantic web), *Necropolitics of Vaccine Capitalism* by Salla

Sariola (visualization of economic differences in global vaccine distribution in the form of data situated on a map), *Sonification of UK Covid Deaths* by Jamie Perera (experimental sonification of statistics from specific time ranges of daily COVID-19 mortality in the United Kingdom). The platform also included other forms using the logic of visualization, therefore making visible issues that have become less visible during the pandemic and definitely more difficult to visually homogenize within top-down commercial infographic strategies, for example: *The Confluence of Institutional Violence and Structural Poverty in Low-Income Neighborhoods of Argentina* by Silvia Hirsch, Andrea Mastrangelo (an anthropological research report on the mutual determinants between structural poverty, physical and symbolic violence and the spread of the virus, which includes ethnographic data, timelines, maps, media resources, among other things), *COVID-19 Propaganda in China* by Margaret Siu (a critical discussion with examples of Chinese COVID-19 political propaganda posters). Just these few examples allow us to conclude that *Visualizing the Virus* is a vast and transdisciplinary platform that does not propose any unified or even averaged perception of the pandemic through different forms of visualization. Moreover, the term *visualization* itself has a much wider scope of meaning here and does not necessarily refer only to graphic forms; it transpires that articles, reports, podcasts and interviews can be equally powerful tools for revealing the underexposed issues we have encountered during the pandemic. Thus, visualization has a more extensive meaning here: it is impossible to read the projects collected on *Visualizing the Virus* separately. It is only as an open, dynamic and fluctuating collection that they begin to take on significance; it is through the 'data friction' mentioned by Loukissas that a deeper understanding of pandemicity is produced in relation to biopolitics, necropolitics, capitalism, economic violence, social problems and the intercultural qualities of media discourse.

It can be said with certainty that *Visualizing the Virus* is an example of curated data: navigation through the collected visualizations is possible in several ways – through the 'Index' function that allows browsing all the projects in alphabetical or chronological order, through contributors, or through 'clusters' – divided into 'themed clusters' that collect visualizations on specific issues, and 'curated clusters' – that allow one to access the data in a transversal way (see Figure 8.2).[5] Curated clusters offer non-obvious forms of narration that reveal hidden meanings emerging from the juxtaposition of individual visualizations. Among the curated clusters, we find such collections as: *White Privilege and COVID-19* (curated by Katherine Blouin, Girish Daswani), *Visualising COVID-19 as a Zoonotic Disease* (curated by Christos Lynteris), *Covid Denialism* (curated by Camelia Dewan, Nicholas Loubere) and *Can't Touch This: Covid19 in the Context of Protests in Hong Kong* (curated by Angela Su). Both the individual visualizations and the construction of the interface itself make critical reference to the methods of automatic visualization

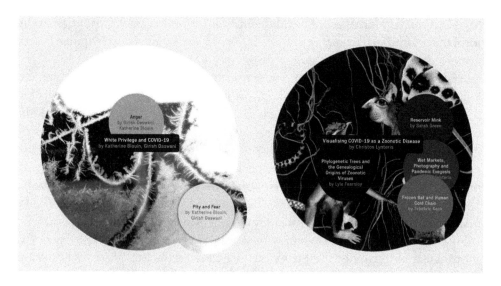

FIGURE 8.2: Visualizing the virus, curated clusters, screenshot from 10 May 2022.

with dots. As we can read in the introduction on the website, 'Through curated clusters and themed clusters that make connections between issues and geographical spaces, *Visualizing the Virus* aims to provide a granular, intersectional picture of the pandemic as it evolves' (Chatterjee 2020: n. pag.). The animated interface does not homogenize the strategy; on the contrary, it increases the friction that emerges between the different themes and visualization methods – in this way, the data are not neutralized in the process of 'expert' narration. It is the viewer's ethical imperative to co-create the narrative and produce responsible knowledge about the pandemic, which, in this case, is not just an epidemic phenomenon; it also contains elements of biopolitical violence, economic pressure and social, racial and cultural inequalities.

Conclusion

As early as June 2020, in the first phase of the pandemic, researchers from the Department of Clinical Pharmacology in Mumbai, observing the reality around them, wrote that:

> In this pandemic, it is very important to engage with the community to improve public trust, help improve design and conduct studies that are responsive to the community's health needs. […] Failure to build and maintain community trust during

the process of research design and implementation, or when disclosing preliminary results, will not only impede study recruitment and completion but may also undermine the uptake of any interventions proven to be efficacious.

(Thatte and Gogtay 2020: 11)

Crises, such as the COVID-19 pandemic, teach us that engaging with affected communities before, during and after a study is essential for building and maintaining trust in science. There cannot be an implementation phase that is separate from designing and conducting research; it has to be a co-creative process. This is how a model of trust in the research itself and its effects is generated (Sulik et al. 2021). Data visualization – as a process of taking data, analysing them, arranging them into sets and representing them in a certain way – is an example that can be used to think about the epistemic gap between science and societies. Kim, Rainecke and Hullman, in their article 'Explaining the gap: Visualizing one's predictions improves recall and comprehension of data' argue that users' initial knowledge of data visualization, and the preconceptions, perceptions and expectations with which they approach the deployment of these processes, should be central to the development of visualization strategies (Kim et al. 2017). Working with the recipients of these visualizations can provide a basis for reducing the epistemic gap through processes of semi-projection and translation (Kim et al. 2018). As Jessica Hullman highlights, there is also a need to communicate the uncertainty involved in the data visualization process (Hullman 2019). This aspect was also pointed out by the researchers at MIT who analysed the visualizations made by anti-maskers, concluding:

Researchers often do not believe that people will understand and be able to interpret results that communicate uncertainty (which, as we have shown, is a problematic assumption at best). However, visualization researchers also do not have a robust body of understanding about how, and when, to communicate uncertainty (let alone how to do so effectively).

(Lee et al. 2021: 16)

The pandemic has shown that the problem of the epistemic gap does not concern the scientists themselves, who are perfectly capable of formulating such doubts. After all, there is a well-established tradition of research among historians, anthropologists and geographers, who have long shown that visualizations – far from objective representations of knowledge – are often, in fact, representations of power (Lee et al. 2021: 3). This problem became apparent elsewhere in the process: in the relationship and interaction between the scientific project and society. Thus, it revealed the need not only for new inter- and transdisciplinary practices but also collective ones which would integrate users from the beginning of the process. Thus, for the process to be changed, it no longer suffices to rely on the interpreter function as a strategy developed within science communication. If visualization is to continue developing to such an extent within data-driven knowledge production, this will generate the need to teach new knowledge-creation skills from the early years of education, not just within the disciplines that are currently responsible for data visualization projects. However, this teaching should include a broader understanding of the process within the socially and historically situated nature of visualization procedures and highlight from the outset the limitations and shortcomings inherent in the tool. It therefore amounts to an epistemic error to socially communicate an objective, truth-generating approach that is based on the immutable certainty of results and their interpretation. This does not mean, however, that it is not helpful in many aspects of society and in diagnosing particular problems. Situating data, working from the bottom up with audience participation, defining mechanisms for data analysis and being critical of various forms of data aggregation and homogenization that cause ethnic, racial, economic and social exclusions can be a good starting point for developing representative and equitable visualization practices and ways of teaching them. This will, perhaps, also allow us to avoid the platformization that visualizations have undergone in the strategies of hijacking visuality and the methods of generating it by groups that deny the reality of the effects of the pandemic.

Analysing the wide range of data visualization strategies that emerged during the pandemic, Alan McConchie – in a blog post in February 2021 entitled *Visualizing the Pulse of a Pandemic: A Year of Covid Line Charts* – identified a number of elements and visualization strategies that have proved helpful, in particular those that treated data as deeply situated and localized and which showed the effects of the virus on a smaller scale. The entry concludes with this important summary:

> As a data visualization community, we have also learned how much we don't know, and still have yet to learn about our tools, our data, and our practice. We also hope that this experience of living through this pandemic year and in our own small or large ways being part of the crisis that is the subject of our charts – of being both the visualizer and the visualized – will give us more sensitivity the next time we find ourselves making visualizations of some crisis or disaster. Dataviz can be humanizing, and dehumanizing, and hopefully this year we've used it not as a distraction from feeling, but as a way to cope through more connection, sensitivity, and understanding.
> (McConchie 2021b: n.pag.)

The lesson learned from data visualization during the pandemic is that there is a risk that in pursuit of predictions and statistics, our data-hungry society will be fed rapid and compulsive visualizations, which can result in the systemic exclusion of problems that do not fit into the mathematical modelling and visualizations developed in accordance with the prevailing standards. As McConchie mentions, sensitivity and connection require rethinking these modalities and introducing new solutions, such as those proposed by the two very different ways of visualizing data discussed in this text, namely, the projects from the Critical Media Lab in Basel and the Collective for Open Data Distribution-Keralam. No doubt there are other examples of data visualization that could be cited, but it is doubtful that any have had such a strong influence on public opinion as the American projects of Johns Hopkins University or the *New York Times*. While appreciating their general perspective on the number of illnesses and deaths on a global scale, it should be noted that they do not take into account the many significant problems that the virus has generated, in terms of mortality of individuals, its effects on entire communities or the deepening poverty affecting specific social groups, which is evident in the lack of access to medical care for indigenous peoples in the Amazon or the limited and expensive distribution of vaccines to African countries. All these phenomena associated with the pandemic actually show that it is a sphere for the distribution of new forms of violence, biopolitics, exploitation and the acceleration of economic and social inequalities. Data visualizations are not neutral ways of showing trends, phenomena and facts; they are aesthetic representations that demand reworking and rethinking in terms of our data-driven society and the new problems that have emerged with the pandemic. Above all, however, they are underexposed areas of violence that still need to be made visible.

ACKNOWLEDGEMENTS

This text is the result of research conducted under the auspices of grants from the Polish Ministry of Education and Science, entitled *Mediated Environments. New Practices in Humanities and Transdisciplinary Research* (no: 0014/NPRH4/H2b/83/2016).

NOTES

1. I finished this text in April 2022, when some countries, mostly European, announced 'the end of pandemia'. But in many places in the world, people were still suffering from infections, and pandemia was far from the end. As human geographer Danny Dorling wrote on the 12 April 2022: 'Far too many think the pandemic is over – or at least coming to an end. The prevalence rates revealed by the various surveillance surveys negate that' (Dorling 2022).
2. https://coronavirus.jhu.edu/map.html. Accessed 22 February 2022.

3. https://covid19kerala.info/. Accessed 22 February 2022.
4. Project website *Visualizing the Virus*: https://visualizingthevirus.com https://criticalmedialab.ch/projects/visualizing-the-virus/. Accessed 22 February 2022.
5. https://visualizingthevirus.com/cluster/. Accessed 22 February 2022.

REFERENCES

Anderson, Marta (2022), 'So many "virologists" in this thread! Impoliteness in Facebook discussions of the management of the pandemic of Covid-19 in Sweden – the tension between conformity and distinction', *Pragmatics*, 32:4, October, pp. 489–517, https://doi.org/10.1075/prag.21014.and.

Atherton, Rachel (2021), '"Missing/Unspecified": Demographic data visualization during the COVID-19 pandemic', *Journal of Business and Technical Communication*, 35:1, pp. 80–87, https://doi.org/10.1177/1050651920957982.

Cairo, Alberto (@AlbertoCairo) (2020), 'This map shows data at various levels of aggregation', Twitter, 12 April, https://twitter.com/AlbertoCairo/status/1249313235955855361. Accessed 20 February 2022.

Callaghan, Sarah (2020), 'COVID-19 is a data science issue', *Patterns*, 1:2, May, https://doi.org/10.1016/j.patter.2020.100022.

Chan, Aileen Lai-yam, Leung, Chi Chiu, Lam, Tai Hing and Cheng, Kar Keung (2020), 'To wear or not to wear: WHO's confusing guidance on masks in the Covid-19 pandemic', *The BMJ Opinion*, 11 March, https://blogs.bmj.com/bmj/2020/03/11/whos-confusing-guidance-masks-covid-19-epidemic/. Accessed 22 February 2022.

Chatterjee, Sria (2020), 'Visualizing the Virus. About the project', https://visualizingthevirus.com/about/. Accessed 22 February 2022.

Coeckelbergh, Mark (2020), 'The postdigital in pandemic times: A comment on the Covid-19 crisis and its political epistemologies', *Postdigital Science and Education*, 2/2020, pp. 547–50, https://doi.org/10.1007/s42438-020-00119-2.

Comba, João L. D. (2020), 'Data visualization for the understanding of COVID-19', *Computing in Science & Engineering*, 22:6, pp. 81–86, November–December, https://doi.org/10.1109/MCSE.2020.3019834.

Dong, Ensheng, Du, Hongru and Gardner, Lauren (2020), 'An interactive web-based dashboard to track COVID-19 in real time', *Lancet Infectious Diseases*, 20, pp. 533–34, https://doi.org/10.1016/S1473-3099(20)30120-1.

Dorling, Danny (2022), 'The never-ending pandemia', *Social Europe*, 12 April, https://socialeurope.eu/the-never-ending-pandemic. Accessed 20 February 2022.

Finn, Ed (2017), *What Algorithms Want? Imagination in the Age of Computing*, Cambridge: MIT Press.

Foucault, Michel (2008), *The Birth of Biopolitics: Lectures at the Collège de France* (trans. M. Senellart), London: Palgrave Macmillan.

Fuchs, Christian (2021), *Communicating COVID-19. Everyday Life, Digital Capitalism, and Conspiracy Theories in Pandemic Times*, Bingley: Emerald.

Gitelman, Lisa (ed.) (2013), *'Raw Data' Is an Oxymoron*, Cambridge: MIT Press.

Hullman, Jessica (2019), 'Confronting unknowns: How to read common visualizations of uncertainty', *Scientific American*, 1 September, https://www.scientificamerican.com/article/how-to-get-better-at-embracing-unknowns/. Accessed 15 February 2022.

Kim, Yea-Seul, Rainecke, Katharina and Hullman, Jessica (2017), 'Explaining the gap: Visualizing one's predictions improves recall and comprehension of data', *Proceedings of the 2017 CHI Conference on Human Factors in Computing Systems (CHI '17)*, New York: Association for Computing Machinery, pp. 1375–86, https://doi.org/10.1145/3025453.3025592.

Kim, Yea-Seul, Rainecke, Katharina and Hullman, Jessica (2018), 'Data through others' eyes: The impact of visualizing others' expectations on visualization interpretation, *IEEE Transactions on Visualization and Computer Graphics*, 24:1, pp. 760–69, https://doi.org/10.1109/TVCG.2017.2745240.

Lee, Crystal, Yang, Tanya, Inchoco, Gabrielle, Jones, Graham M. and Satyanarayan, Arvind (2021), 'Viral visualizations: How Coronavirus skeptics use orthodox data practices to promote unorthodox science online', *Proceedings of the 2021 CHI Conference on Human Factors in Computing Systems*, Yokohama: Association for Computing Machinery, May, https://doi.org/10.1145/3411764.3445211.

Loukissas, Yanni Alexander (2019), *All Data Are Local: Thinking Critically in a Data-Driven Society*, Cambridge, MA: MIT Press.

McConchie, Alan (2021a), *Corona-Cartography: What We Learned from a Year of COVID-19 Maps*, https://medium.com/hi-stamen/corona-cartography-what-we-learned-from-a-year-of-covid-19-maps-bd1f022bc5e0. Accessed 10 March 2022.

McConchie, Alan (2021b), 'Visualizing the pulse of a pandemic: A year of COVID line charts' *Stamen*, 25 March, https://stamen.com/visualizing-the-pulse-of-a-pandemic-a-year-of-covid-line-charts-52368b4a22b0/. Accessed 10 March 2022.

Michie, Jonathan (2020), 'The degeneration of capitalism from a system of production to a speculative orgy', *International Review of Applied Economics*, 34:2, pp. 147–51, https://doi.org/10.1080/02692171.2020.1720164.

Milner, Greg (2020), 'Creating the dashboard for the pandemic', *ArcUser*, Summer, pp. 56–59, https://www.esri.com/about/newsroom/wp-content/uploads/2020/08/jhu_dashboard.pdf. Accessed 20 February 2022.

Parikka, Jussi (2007), *Digital Contagions: A Media Archaeology of Computer Viruses*, New York: Peter Lang.

Sulik, Justin, Deroy, Ophelia, Dezecache, Guillaume, Newson, Martha, Zhao, Yi, El Zein, Marwa and Tunçgenç, Bahar (2021), 'Facing the pandemic with trust in science', *Humanities and Social Sciences Communications*, 8:301, pp. 1–10, https://doi.org/10.1057/s41599-021-00982-9.

Sundaram, Ravi (2021), '"Response," Sundaram, Ravi, Terranova, Tiziana, "Colonial infrastructues and techno-social networks"', *e-flux*, December, 123, http://worker01.e-flux.com/pdf/article_437385.pdf. Accessed 15 February 2022.

Ulahannan, Jijo Pulickiyil, Narayanan, Nikhil, Thalhath, Nishad, Prabhakaran, Prem, Chaliyeduth, Sreekanth, Suresh, Sooraj P, Mohammed, Musfir, Rajeevan, E, Sindhu, Joseph, Balakrishnan, Akhil, Uthaman, Jeevan, Karingamadathil, Manoj, Thonikkuzhiyil Sunil Thomas, Sureshkumar, Unnikrishnan, Balan, Shabeesh, Vellichirammal, Neetha Nanoth and the Collective for Open Data Distribution-Keralam (CODD-K) Consortium (2020), 'A citizen science initiative for open data and visualization of COVID-19 outbreak in Kerala, India', *Journal of the American Medical Informatics Association*, 27:12, pp. 1913–20, https://doi.org/10.1093/jamia/ocaa203.

Thatte, Urmilla M. and Gogtay, Nithya J. (2020), 'Research and ethics during the COVID-19 pandemic', *Journal of the Association of India*, 68, pp. 11–12, https://www.japi.org/v2c474b4/research-and-ethics-during-the-covid-19-pandemic. Accessed 22 February 2022.

9

How Language Conceptualized the Pandemic

Małgorzata Majewska

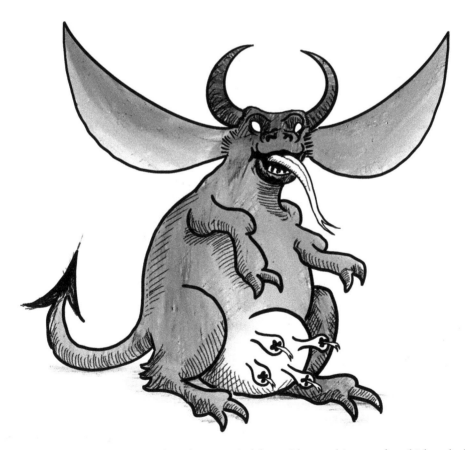

FIGURE 9.1: Cartoon representing what our mind does with something new for which we lack the language. Courtesy of Maciek Dziadyk.

Famine, pestilence and war have never left the first places of humankind's priorities. Successive generations prayed to all sorts of gods, holy angels, invented innumerable tools, institutions and social systems – and yet people still died en masse of starvation, epidemics and violence. Therefore, many thinkers and prophets have concluded that famine, pestilence and war are simply an integral part of God's cosmic plan, or possibly our imperfect nature. […] At the dawn of the third millennium, humanity realizes […] that in the last few decades we have managed to curb famine, pestilence and war.

(Harari 2018: 8)

It wasn't that bad yet. The world is full of diseases that we didn't even hear about two decades ago! A few rich people own as much wealth as the poorer half of humanity. From the screens and columns we are shocked by the information about bloody wars and millions of refugees, about increasingly sophisticated tortures and terrorist attacks. As if that wasn't enough, new technologies enable surveillance at every turn and the production of devilishly effective propaganda. Plague, famine, wars and captivity. We live in an apocalypse. We encounter prophets announcing it every step of the way […] Unfortunately, all of these claims are true. We are constantly attacked by new diseases; there are places in the world where people starve to death, are murdered or are in captivity. And yet – we live in the best times. The world has never been so healthy and full, so safe and free. This is not wishful thinking, but the result of an analysis of data in the field of medicine, economy, military history and political history.

(Napiórkowski 2017: 'Tygodnik Powszechny', No. 37/2017)

These two quotations are taken from two very different sources. The first is drawn from Yuval Harari's book *Homo Deus: A Brief History of Tomorrow*. The second is drawn from Polish semiotician Marcin Napiórkowski's article 'We live in the best times'. At the time that these words were written, no one knew the word *Covid* and no one knew that another war would break out – this time in Ukraine. However, drawing on ideas from these texts, I want to explore how people dealt with and are continuing to deal with the pandemic today. To do this, I adopt a perceptual-linguistic perspective and methodological tools proposed by cognitive linguistics as a way of analysing language and meaning. My general thesis assumes that humans, when faced with a new experience, need to give it meaning and the way they do that is expressed in language. To illustrate this idea, I analysed selected language structures that appeared in the Polish media during the pandemic (2020–21). From a perceptual point of view, the media's framing of the pandemic required a new category related to the medical domain, which in turn triggered a sense of agency and responsibility, and not – as before – external control, which was understood as delegating responsibility to gods or higher forces.

Examples similar to Harari or Napiórkowski quoted above are all around us. When something traumatic happens, our perception has to tame it somehow. If we have a conceptual grid ready for it, we enter a new event into it. If what has happened does not yet have a narrative, i.e. a conceptual grid, then our minds immediately go to work. And, with the help of the two most important cognitive mechanisms – metaphor and metonymy – we tame what we experience. The results of this familiarization are recorded in language.

When encountering COVID-19, I suggest that people face the pandemic not medically but perceptually-linguistically. Here, I adopt the perspective assumed by cognitive linguistics, which assumes that 'the study of language is the study of the processes of human cognition' (Tabakowska 2011: 199). I analysed language constructions that appeared in the Polish media during the pandemic, i.e. from 11 March 2020, when the director general of the World Health Organization, Tedros Adhanom Ghebreyesus, described the development of the disease as a pandemic. By May 16, the regulation of the Minister of Health abolished the state of epidemic in Poland that had been in force since 20 March 2020 and replaced it with a state of epidemic emergency (Polish Press Association 2022).

Due to the limited scope of this chapter, my analyses are qualitative and aim to demonstrate examples of pandemic conceptualization. The research sample is too small to be a statistical study; however, I consider it sufficient to reinforce the thesis that, in the face of a new experience, people need to give it meaning and the way they do this will be expressed in language. To illustrate this, I begin with a necessary cognitive thesis, which will form the basis for the presented linguistic analyses, as I seek to examine what meaning Polish-language users gave to the pandemic. I present and analyse the most common constructions and metaphors in order to test Harari's hypothesis, which was put forward before the SARS-CoV-2 virus appeared in the world. From a perceptual point of view, Harari assumes that the current way of taming or getting to grips with a pandemic – at the level of the semantic scheme – consists of the internal triggering of a sense of agency and responsibility, and not – as before – of a form of external control, which was understood as delegating responsibility to gods or higher forces.

Theoretical assumptions

In western cultural circles, it was assumed for a long time, following Aristotle, that language objectively describes the existing world. This objectivist model of viewing the world minimized the role of an individual language user and sought universal, objectified meanings. George Lakoff, in the introduction to the now classic book on meaning in language entitled *Women, Fire and Dangerous Things*, defines these differences in language, dividing them into traditional and experiential. The traditional (objectivist) approach to language means that:

> The mind is abstract and separate from the body. [A person] sees the mind as literal, operating mainly on propositions that are either objectively true or objectively false [...] The ability to reason is abstract and need not be ingrained in the organism. Meaningful concepts and rational thought are therefore transcendent in the sense that they transcend the physical limits of the organism. Meaningful concepts and abstract reason may reside in man, or in machine, or in some other organism – but their existence is abstract, independent of concrete embodiment.
>
> (Lakoff 2011: 6)

The experiential approach to language is based on empirical research; essentially, it deprives language of its objective character and transfers it to the shaky ground of uncertainty, subjectivity and what might be considered unscientific. According to Lakoff:

> The new view gives centrality to the imaginative aspects of reason – metaphor, metonymy and mental imagery – which have hitherto been regarded as peripheral, irrelevant appendages to the literal. [...] Meaning is related to what is meaningful to thinking living beings.
>
> (2011: 8)

The experiential model assumes that 'language is one of several human cognitive abilities, so its description must refer to human categorization abilities or the ability to direct attention to a selected element of reality and isolate it from the background' (Langacker 2009: 7). Therefore, we assume that language shows the speaker's way of seeing reality and the role they assign to themselves in this perception. This assumption meets the belief that people tame reality by giving it meaning, and not – as assumed in the objectivist model – by discovering it.

Our perception needs to find some order in the chaos of events, the key to understanding and sometimes making sense of what is happening. Humans, looking for the order of the world, deceive themselves that by discovering single scientific laws, they will discover the same laws concerning, for example, the meaning of death or suffering. There is a danger of erroneous assumptions that the world has this internal order and that we are able to discover it. Meanwhile, the search for order gives us a sense of control and security, but this feeling lasts until there is an element or event that will violate or even negate this order (e.g. a borderline experience).

This assumption of cognitive linguistics is grounded in philosophy. In her book *Tożsamość i różnica* (Skarga 1997) – or *Identity and Difference* – Barbara Skarga indicates that the lack of identity would put us in front of a world of chaos, senseless things and events appearing, absolute changeability, in which we ourselves would dissolve from the inside in a stream of disordered impressions, without a point of support, like a current changing. As long as people express themselves in the world and have a sense of agency (i.e. influence on this world), they introduce their own order to it or realize themselves by connecting the self to the intersubjectively defined order of the world. Identity in given areas provides a sense of belonging, anchoring in some reality.

So, we look for similarities between what new things are happening around us in addition to known and recognizable events. In other words, we are looking for a category into which a new experience can be entered. The ability to categorize allows us to function in the world. For most of us, experiencing a pandemic on such a scale was something new that we could not describe due to the lack of a mental scheme for such a situation.

Each new situation needs to create its own narrative. It used to be produced by interlocutors in everyday relationships. Today, this burden has been partially taken over by the media, including social media. These narratives were analysed as part of interdisciplinary research conducted by the Institute of Journalism of the Jagiellonian University and the Institute of Psychology as part of the grant 'How to inform so as not to traumatise? Journalistic and psychological aspects of media coverage of the COVID-19 pandemic.' The grant was financed by the SocietyNow!#1 competition under the Strategic Programme. For the purposes of this chapter, it is worth taking a closer look at these narratives from a linguistic point of view, looking not only at their overall message but also at individual linguistic elements showing the most important thing for us: the extent to which taming the COVID-19 pandemic triggers agency and the extent to which – how in the old days – it was moved to the space outside the zone of action, to the space beyond control, attributing responsibility for pandemics to magical powers or divine action. Importantly, the pandemic had no concrete images. There was no rash or any other distinguishing sign that might have been the basis for conceptualizing the virus.

In particular, the narrative concerns information that may arouse or increase the level of fear among recipients in a way that is inappropriate or disproportionate to the situation. Of course, many fears in this particular situation were justified and could lead to positive results, for example, increased caution in situations of exposure to infection, or more careful protection of oneself and others, mutual assistance and care, and compliance with regulations and restrictions. However, arousing excessive fear that is inadequate to the situation or based on

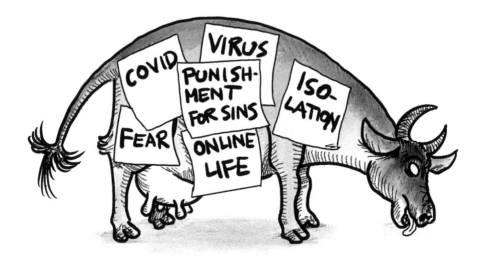

FIGURE 9.2: Cartoon representing how we tame difficult words through language. When something that scares us gets a name, we have the false sense that we can somehow control it. Courtesy of Maciek Dziadyk.

untrue premises can have potentially negative social consequences, as well as be counterproductive – instead of sensitizing to threats and provoking reflection, protective measures are rejected in the belief that one way or another they don't matter (Całek et al. 2022: 11).

According to the cited study, which was based on media materials that provided the basis for information and narrative construction, in the spring of 2020, seven thematic areas aroused the greatest anxiety or fear among Poles in the first quarter of lockdown.

The first is medical information. Yes, the virus itself was new, but our conceptual system had a ready-made conceptual grid. The project analyses it in detail in relation to another disease discussed by Susan Sontag in her book *Illness as a Metaphor* (1978). The next themes are the problems of the health service, the individual experience of the epidemic and its personal costs for individuals – political, administrative and legal matters. Next are the causes of the epidemic – prognoses and forecasts for the future and figures (Całek et al. 2022: 33–38). In this chapter, selected examples of conceptual mixtures that have appeared in the media will be shown.

> While dogs, cats, horses, and other familiar species presumably must do perceptual binding of the sort needed to see a single dog, cat, or horse, human beings are exceptionally adept at integrating two extraordinarily different inputs to create new

emergent structures, which result in new tools, new technologies, and new ways of thinking.

(Fauconnier 2002: 27)

Our minds invisibly and unconsciously organize an extensive conceptual network, thanks to which we can mentally, within this network, experience emotions and take part in scenarios that are inaccessible through real experience. Such a construction of conceptual mixtures is later referred to as mental spaces.

When lockdown was introduced in the first phase of the pandemic, journalist Danuta Pawłowska, in the article 'Coronavirus in the world. State at the end of 2020', created the following mental space: 'In Poland today there is supposed to be a "supposed curfew" and from 7 p.m. on the last day of the year to 6 a.m. on January 1, we are not to move' (Pawłowska 2020: n.pag.). The mix here has two contributions: the coronavirus and the socio-state related to the curfew. The content projection into the mixture is only partial. In this case, the speaker only borrowed the timeframe prohibiting citizens from leaving their homes. In contrast, the reasons for the ban on this mixture already come from the coronavirus contribution.

The following text appeared on the Medicover website:

Coronavirus 2020 – a year marked by a pandemic

The end of the year is approaching, so it's time to sum up. Unfortunately, 2020 has been hard on everyone. The pandemic caused by the novel coronavirus has turned our world upside down and is still taking its toll. However, there is a glimmer of hope, scientists have probably developed an effective vaccine. So let's not break down – the new year is a new page, but before we open it, let's summarize what has changed this year.[1]

The second area of the contribution, next to the Covid contribution, is the agricultural contribution, because the pandemic is taking its toll. Thanks to this, a mental space is created that triggers thinking about the virus as something that was once planted like a seed. It has had time to mature, and now it is time to harvest. Interestingly, in the basic agricultural sense, this idiom appears together with a positive valuation. The bigger the harvest, the more bountiful the harvest, the better. Here, the negative connotation in the mental space is borrowed from the disease input and triggers negative valuing. In other words, the greater the toll of the pandemic, the worse it becomes.

In the same sentence, Covid, as the factor that caused the pandemic, is indicated as being responsible for turning our world upside down. It is not magical powers or God, as was the case in the old days, that are pointed to as responsible, but the coronavirus. On the other hand, the noun *pandemic* launches a conceptualization that indicates the mass nature of its impact. It is worth noting the possessive pronoun *our* combined with the noun *world*, which indicates that the virus is perceived as something external to our sphere of influence. It is this external factor that threatens us, so this factor must be eliminated. In another text, Dr Paweł Grzesiowski, president of the Institute of Infection Prevention Foundation, stated in an interview published in *Gazeta Wyborcza* on 6 April 2020 that the virus attacks. This is a mental space in which the virus is a conscious entity and, at the same time, an enemy, so it must be fought.

Meningitis and encephalitis are not a disease that is specifically related to the virus. The virus attacks mainly the respiratory tract, possibly the circulatory system.[2] Nowadays, we often do not attribute the threat of death to some metaphysical mystery. Rather, we conceptualize it as a defined problem that needs to be solved. Here, the solution is a vaccine, which is a ray of hope. The language here shows a mental space that is made up of two inputs: medical and weather-related imagery. In the weather cartridge, a ray is an element of the sun that warms the world. In the mental space, it is an element of hope that, like the sun, warms us with the thought of solving the problem of the pandemic.

Once upon a time, death was seen differently:

Medieval fairy tales depicted death as a hooded figure in a black cloak, holding a great scythe. A man lives a normal life, and suddenly a grim reaper appears in front of him, pokes him on the shoulder with a bony finger and says: 'Come!'. Then the man pleads with her, 'No, please! Give me another year, month, day!' But the hooded figure whistles back, 'No. You must come with me NOW!'.

(Harari 2018: 33)

Today, it is thrown into a cause-and-effect scheme. That's why Harari says: no other route of infection has been confirmed other than droplet and mucosal transmission. The medical domain was the most powerful interpretative framework. Hence, the common use of terms from its semantic area: symptoms, disease, course, route of infection, severity of disease symptoms and disinfection. It was in this domain that the taming of the pandemic in the twenty-first century took place. Thanks to this, the causative aspect was strongly activated because the mental scheme assumed that it was a virus, and viruses can be fought, so finding a cure is simply a matter of time. The vaccine narrative was created before specific vaccines were introduced to the general public.

According to the cited studies conducted by media experts and psychologists, media narratives triggered anxiety in the recipients, but it was still maintained in the causative conceptualization because it was based on the effects of medicine.

In summary, conventional conceptualization is the process by which new information is compared with previous experiences and existing, conventionalized language phrases are recalled. Meanwhile, the experience of the pandemic was so new that it required the creation of a new conceptualization, i.e. a new language. For me, the issue of agency was particularly important. To what extent our perception of the pandemic was based on mental patterns, emphasizing our passivity towards the disease, and to what extent our responsibility for it and the ability to fight it? It remains to be hoped that the created conceptual categories will not be needed and that COVID-19 is a one-time experience.

NOTES

1. *Polish version: Koronawirus 2020 – czyli rok pod znakiem pandemii Zbliża się koniec roku, czas więc na podsumowania. Niestety rok 2020 dał się wszystkim mocno we znaki. Pandemia wywołana przez nowego koronawirusa **postawiła nasz świat na głowie i wciąż zbiera swe żniwo**. Pojawił się jednak promyk nadziei, naukowcy opracowali prawdopodobnie skuteczną szczepionkę. Nie załamujmy się zatem – nowy rok to nowa karta, ale zanim ją otworzymy podsumujmy, co się zmieniło w tym roku.*
2. *https://wyborcza.pl/7,82983,25848418,koronawirus-czy-wszyscy-zachorujemy-czy-jest-lek-ktory-dziala.html. Accessed 30 April 2024. Polish version: Akurat zapalenie opon mózgowo-rdzeniowych i mózgu nie jest chorobą, która w jakiś szczególny sposób wiąże się z wirusem. Wirus atakuje głównie drogi oddechowe, ewentualnie układ krążenia.*

REFERENCES

Bryła, Władysława and Bryła-Cruz, Agnieszka (2021), *Retoryka okołokoronawirusowa. Szkice językowo-kulturowe*, Lublin: UMCS.

Całek, Agnieszka, Hodalska, Magdalena and Małgorzata, Lisowska-Magdziarz (2022), *Covid, Media i Lęk. Informacje o epidemii Covid-19 jako czynnik zwiększający społeczny niepokój i poczucie zagrożenia*, Cracow: Jagiellonian University, p. 11.

Fauconnier, Gilles (2002), *Mental Spaces: Aspects of Meaning Construction in Natural Language*, Cambridge: Cambridge University Press.

Harari, Yuval N. ([2015] 2018), *Homo Deus: A Brief History of Tomorrow (trans. M. Romanek)*, Kraków: Wydawnictwo Literackie

Lakoff, George (2011), *Women, Fire and Dangerous Things: What Categories Tell Us About the Mind* (ed. E. Tabakowska, trans. M. Buchta, A. Kotarba and A. Skucińska), Cracow: Universitas.

Langacker, Ronald W. (2009), *Cognitive Grammar: Introduction (przeł. Zespół)*, Cracow: Universitas.

Medicover websites, https://www.medicover.pl/koronawirus/. Accessed 24 March 2023.

Napiórkowski, Marcin (2017), 'Tygodnik Powszechny', No. 37/2017.

Pawłowska, Danuta (2020), 'Koronawirus na świecie. Stan na koniec 2020 r.', *Gazeta Wyborcza*, 31 December, https://biqdata.wyborcza.pl/biqdata/7,159116,26651431,koronawirus-na-swiecie-stan-na-koniec-2020-r.html. Accessed 25 March 2023.

Polish Press Association (2022), 'Kiedy koniec stanu zagrożenia epidemicznego w Polsce? Minister Niedzielski mówi jasno', *MedOnet*, 6 December, https://www.medonet.pl/koronawirus/koronawirus-w-polsce,kiedy-koniec-stanu-zagrozenia-epidemicznego-w-polsce--minister-niedzielski-mowi-jasno,artykul,87019952.html. Accessed 25 March 2023.

Roman, Dorota (2020), Interview with Paweł Grzesiowski. 'Gazeta Wyborcza', 6 April, https://wyborcza.pl/7,82983,25848418,koronawirus-czy-wszyscy-zachorujemy-czy-jest-lek-ktory-dziala.html. Accessed 24 March 2023.

Skarga, Barbara (1997), *Tożsamość i różnica: eseje metafizyczne*, Krakow: Wydawnictwo Znak.

Sontag, Susan (1978), *Illness as Metaphor*, New York: Farrar, Straus & Giroux.

Tabakowska, Elżbieta (2011), 'W co przechodzi ludzkie pojęcie?' in J. Bremer and A. Chuderski (eds), *Pojęcia. Jak reprezentujemy i kategoryzujemy świat*, Cracow: Universitas. pp. 199–213.

10

Pandemic Discourse: From Intimidation to Social Distancing

Rūta Petrauskaitė and Darius Amilevičius

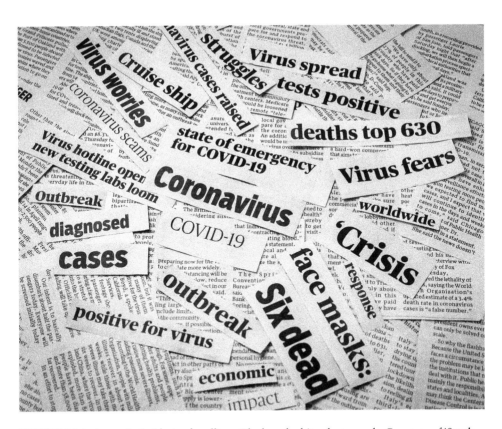

FIGURE 10.1: Anon. *Intimidating headlines*. Black and white photograph. Courtesy of iStock.

Introduction

COVID-19: More than two years of public discourse on the same subject at a variety of levels, through a variety of channels and from a variety of viewpoints. Discourse was developed together with the talked-about events, actions, situations, and their interpretations. Discourse was intended to not only reflect and show something but also to affect and change the course of events. What was this pandemic discourse like? What kind of narrative was constructed in the texts on this topic? How did it change over time? How did it reflect events and people, bearing in mind the fact that, by means of language and of text, by its form and functions and by its connections with other texts, much more is implied than merely transmitted by its content? If one wishes to take up and understand texts in their context, i.e. the whole discourse, the latter must be identified in terms of theme and period, partitioned into stages, and have its most important moments picked out and synthesized so that the entirety of the discourse and its dominant tendencies become evident. That is what we shall do, confining our attention to two years, dividing this time span into periods that determine the essential ways of speaking on this theme and distinguishing the groups of speakers according to their goals and ideologies, which are recognizable based on their ways and means of expressing themselves.

The object of this research is the Lithuanian pandemic discourse as it occurred in publications during the two years following the start of the first quarantine in the most popular news portals (15min.lt, delfi.lt. lrt.lt., vdu.lt, vz.lt). This discourse was researched by applying the conceptions and approaches of qualitative research methods and using an interpretative approach of critical discourse analysis (Fairclough 1995; Wodak and Meyer 2001). *These approaches were chosen because of their particular interest in the relationship between language and power and in the characterization of 'the Other' and of personalities of another type (as in the old tradition of investigating antisemitic discourse), as well as in their attention to ideology and their interpretation of frameworks that organize sets of attitudes, and especially because of their attention to the formal side of the texts, their language, style, stereotypes and implications. Quantitative methods were used to extract keywords and key phrases (bigrams and trigrams) from the headlines of relevant texts of each pandemic period, which made up a word cloud. Despite the use of quantitative methods, this article concentrates on the evaluative aspect; therefore, we will begin by presenting the evaluative connotations of an otherwise neutral genre, that of information-bearing reports,* and these connotations become evident in the titles of the reports. Later, when discussing the evaluative genre itself, we will limit ourselves to the so-called mainstream news portals, and we will mention the discourse peculiar to social media only to the extent that its reflections also occur in mainstream portals.

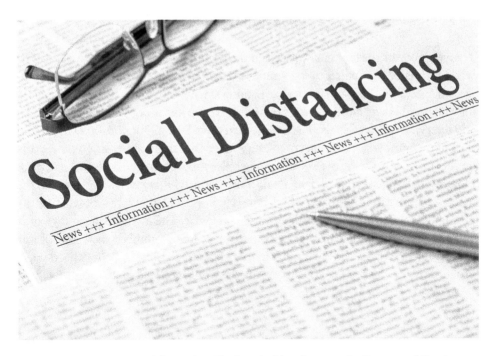

FIGURE 10.2: Anon. *Social distancing*. Black and white photograph. Courtesy of iStock.

The COVID-19 period in Lithuania is divided into pandemic waves and events associated with them: quarantines (the first lasting three months; the second nearly eight), vaccines, the so-called vaccine passport (operative for almost nine months) and public reaction (protests, demonstrations, etc.) to government decisions. Changes in the public discourse do not always coincide with the chronology of pandemic events, which is why this article concentrates on stages in the development of the discourse, especially its connoted level, its evaluative elements and its verbal expression. The goal of this chapter is to review and introduce the dynamics of the discourse, its leading voices and the views they express, looking at the entire discourse from the point of view of its verbal expression. This research makes use of nearly 100 authorized comments on the topic of COVID-19 for a quantitative approach. The qualitative analysis was based on a corpus of approximately 120 thousand headlines that make up more than 845 thousand running words. The presentation here preserves their authentic language so that, in addition to the dialogue of the authors, the different voices of those participating in the discourse might be heard. For this reason, the text contains many citations that illustrate the peculiarities of language and style, which are summarized in the final section.

Intimidating discourse

This stage covers the first quarantine and the beginning of the second, up to the time when Lithuania started receiving vaccines (i.e. it covers the period from March to December 2020). During that time, the mainstream news channels mostly transmitted information-bearing news reports, press releases from institutions of the health system and interviews with officials. The pandemic received the major portion of space and time in the portals since it concerned everyone; particularly important were reports on the statistics showing the numbers of people who were infected, sick or had died. Notably, the statistics were given in absolute numbers that were not relative to the extent of testing, and the causes of death were not detailed in terms of whether the person died while having COVID-19 or died from it. The most frequent keywords and phrases of this period are cases, victims of coronavirus, numbers increased, deaths of COVID-19, crisis, lockdown, COVID-patients, etc. Astrologer Lolita's horoscope/prognoses were at the top of the list during the whole period (see the wordle below).

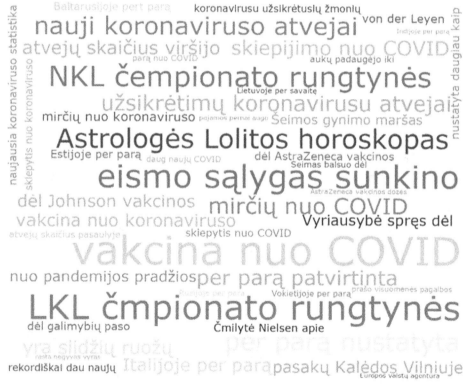

FIGURE 10.3: *A Wordle of Coronavirus* headlines from Lithuanian news portals. Image: Darius Amilevičius.

At the beginning of the quarantine period, texts of information-bearing genres were dominant. Attention must be paid to the titles of the texts, as many people read just those without delving into the texts themselves. Because of their visibility and interpretational nature, titles are treated as separate and almost autonomous brief texts that do not always reflect the essence of the denominated text. A trial investigation of titles in Lithuanian news portals on COVID-19 (Kalinauskaitė and Aleksandravičiūtė-Šviažienė 2020) revealed the dominant functions of titles during the first quarantine and the beginning of the second. In many different news portals, the titles performed the same function – they communicated irritation (66 per cent). This type of communication covers several different aspects that shed light on its nature: dissatisfaction expressed in various forms of anger and its derivatives, lack of safety in the company of other people and the potentially arising danger to medical personnel, problems caused by the coronavirus and quarantine, lack of trust, mutual misunderstanding and fearmongering. The last subgroup is the most numerous (Kalinauskaitė and Aleksandravičiūtė-Šviažienė 2020).

A smaller group (more than 30 per cent) is constituted by subjectively interpreted facts in reports whose titles contain evaluative elements forming a certain attitude towards the topics discussed. These titles seek to hyperbolize: Quarantine in Vilnius: Streams of People Flow in To Spend Free Time (delfi.lt); or to talk about records: Eye of the Storm: The Second COVID-19 Nightmare Has Blown In (15min.lt.); or to exaggerate in other ways, for example, by frequently using the number word Hundreds. The smallest group of titles examined accounts for less than 3 per cent of the total and is intended only to inform: Klaipėda gets its mobile coronavirus testing station (delfi.lt).

The dominant discourse of titles may be described as negative, essentially intended to instil fear. The communication of irritation is incompatible with the principles governing the management of crises in the healthcare system. The most important of these principles calls attention to the fact that 'too large a current of negative information about threats to health can have undesirable effects on people's psychological condition or even mental health' (Kalinauskaitė and Aleksandravičiūtė-Šviažienė 2020: 183). The communication of irritation at different levels of intensity lasted nearly two years, and it only grew weaker when the omicron variety became dominant and government policy substantially changed. Then portals under investigation confined themselves to bare statistics avoiding titles with alarming evaluations although the numbers of COVID-19 at that time were several dozen times bigger in comparison with those in the spring of 2020.

During the spring quarantine of 2020, the first group to reflect on it consisted of public intellectuals who compared it to Camus's *The Plague* and Boccaccio's

Decameron. The philosopher Gintautas Mažeikis (2020a, b) spoke about the relationship between the government and the individual, about the moral judgement to accept the requirements of the quarantine, about the individual's rights to decide whether to be taken over by the state, about the citizens' moral responsibility and about which external forces try to suppress a different opinion that could save the government from making mistakes.

A bit later, the same philosopher (Mažeikis 2020b) reflected on the quarantine's positive aspects of achieving control of borders and the recognition of distance as a token of value and respect that permitted 'the rebirth of civilized, meaningful differences, languages and styles, but not of unbridled tourism and buying sprees'. What's more, the quarantine allowed people to renounce unneeded attributes of contemporary life. 'Understanding the value of walls and distances helps us to comprehend that many things of the "other" life were just unnecessary.' But Mažeikis also recognized the dangers of being closed off:

> The silent loneliness of a domestic quarantine reveals the pitfalls of renouncing a public life, fear of company, the terror of being touched by others and even encourages exaggerated illusions of nationalism, the conviction that walls are more significant than roads.

He consoled himself and others with the thought that 'the rebirth of fences, borders, and a multitude of autonomies encouraged by the crowned virus does not at all mean the end of globalization'.

The summer break from COVID-19 and later the parliamentary elections and the political interregnum somewhat cooled the media frenzy on the pandemic and allowed for the appearance of other subjects. However, in the autumn, the virus reappeared, victim figures doubling in size as the second quarantine commenced, which at first was promised to last three months but in fact lasted nearly eight.

Official commentators scolded the old government (that no longer controlled the situation), which was not prepared for the second pandemic wave and the second quarantine coinciding with the arrival of the new government. A regular commentator who was frightened by a COVID-19 statistic on the night of All Souls' Day spoke of the pandemic's danse macabre, where anyone could infect anyone else and where hospitals are filled beyond capacity. A divide between those who fulfilled the demands of the quarantine and those who tried to evade them became apparent. A deeper reason for this divergence lies in the so-called conspiracy theories or what is attributed to them. In this paper, the term conspiracy theories is used very loosely, without delving into their essence and variety, but treating them more as a way to distinguish those believing in them from those who do not. This divide became a real cause of mutual enmity on social media, and the reflections of this enmity extended even into the most popular news portals.

Here, two discourses become evident: one sceptical of the factors deepening the divide and one keeping it up. The philosopher Nida Vasiliauskaitė (2020b), commenting on the hunt for conspirators on Facebook, revealed its surprising extent and content when all the conspiracy theories were thrown together into one heap. These conspiracies included the following: the Earth is flat, 5G is dangerous, vaccines harm you, the climate isn't getting warmer, the Russians aren't attacking, the politicians are lying to you, US elections were fraudulent, COVID-19 doesn't exist, masks don't help, the world is ruled by reptiles from the Moon, etc. She sarcastically deconstructed the mechanism of making people look stupid, a mechanism allegorically called 'The Knight of Light Pierces the Dragon of Darkness with his Spear of Reason':

> The Sharp Spear of Reason will always in one fell swoop penetrate the whole packet. It just can't be that one who doubts the effectiveness of masking would disbelieve in reptiles and refuse to boil vinegar, that an eye seeing the fall of U.S. democracy wouldn't wink in Russian; that those lacking confidence in the government wouldn't wrap their brainless heads in aluminium foil. Yep, this just can't be – any educated person gets it at once; you can't explain it to the stupid ones; and it just isn't worth wasting your time on this.

Here and elsewhere (17 March 2021), she ironized the destroyers of 'myths' by analysing their texts and exaggerating the opposition between the allegedly enlightened and the non-enlightened. The destroyers do not give any arguments; they just make naive assertions. Moreover, they inadequately present the theories they criticize, answer the wrong questions, rush through open doors and then unconditionally denounce dissidents without first even listening to them. Then, at the end of the text comes a rhetorical question, exposing the destroyers' stupidity: what does the conspiratologist's cement-hard belief in the global conspiracy and its unavoidable success remind you of? Isn't it the conspiratologists themselves? In other words, Vasiliauskaitė shows that those tearing down the myths are not all that different from those believing in them.

A similar discourse was championed by Andrius Jakučiūnas (2020), who described its rhetoric, first dominant on Facebook and then spreading to mainstream media, using a vulgar sports metaphor: 'shittalkers versus pimplenoses – a sorry draw'.

A philosopher already mentioned (Mažeikis 2021) presented his liberal opinion about conspiracy theories and those believing in them. He recommended leaving them in peace because 'once forbidden they will immediately come back strengthened'. Unlike many other commentators, he did not think that it was only uneducated people who believe in conspiracy theories; rather, that such theories are mostly believed in by those who tend towards determinism. At the same time, Mažeikis pathologized believers in conspiracy theories by referring to an alleged claim made by psychiatry that 'too eager a counting of causes and consequences is pathological. A desire to determine the cause of everything is a symptom of sickness – such people draw endless maps, identify secret agencies, black points, Masonic orders'. This tendency also became evident in the texts of other people who considered themselves enlightened, especially the influencers who claimed that conspiracy theories are there to subdue society and make it look stupid. However, by claiming this, they are acting the same way – simulating scientific argumentation or distorting it. According to the philosopher Nida Vasiliauskaitė (2020a), 'almost all mainstream politicians, the advertising industry as well as the normal, non-marginal media are doing the same'.

The topic of vaccination served to antagonize society even more than the conspiracy theories did. Before vaccinations commenced, the mainstream media supported government policy and joined the campaign, urging people to get vaccinated and some columnists were especially active in this regard. However, with the first pandemic year ending, Rimvydas Valatka (2020) remarked that although the government and half of the nation are waiting for the vaccine like it was salvation, the other half will refuse to be vaccinated. He was right in saying that this was just the start of Lithuania's problems. That other half of Lithuania was immediately dubbed antivaxxers, pimplenoses (because they walk around with their mask pushed down below their noses) and idiots because 'the number of brains affected by COVID-19 in Lithuania is greater than the number of lungs'. Then, the charlatans, both named and unnamed, were accused of making Lithuanians seem stupid, while science and medicine 'stand in the corner of the government's reception hall'. Valatka asked, 'What to do? Introduce compulsory vaccination? The answer? Certainly not! This is a free country'. Then he made a suggestion to the Lithuanian government that was not very different from prescribing compulsory vaccination – introduce a vaccine passport similar to a personal identity card or a Lithuanian citizen's passport. Without it, you could not get in anywhere unless the owner of the establishment allowed it. In that case, owners could put up a sign stating, 'Our restaurant, hotel, bus is friendly to cats, dogs, parakeets and antivaxxers.' A similarly mordant irony was put into play by the satirist Juozas Erlickas, who suggested treating antivaxxers like wild African animals – first put them to sleep, then give them the shot. Thus name-calling, insulting, mocking, sarcasm and irony all became marks of public pandemic speaking in Lithuania.

Occasionally, Valatka's discourse became particularly severe and condemnatory. To make life difficult for antivaxxers who believed in the fairy tales of charlatans and spat on scientists' lawns, he suggested that they not only be forced to acquire a vaccine passport but also be required to pay an increased health insurance premium. The arguments for this are based on the perceived rights and duties spelt out in the Constitution, especially the duty to defend the homeland against enemies, one of which, according to the author, is COVID-19. Dealing with this enemy requires a strict policy:

> The essential principle of a liberal democracy states that my and your freedom ends at the point where it begins to infringe on another person's freedom. In this case it is the duty of the state to guarantee that the freedom of the pimplenoses and anti-vaxxers does not interfere with the freedom of a citizen guarding himself and others from the ravages of war, the plague and hunger.

Thus, at the end of 2020, the pandemic discourse, in addition to frightening people, also began to discriminate and marginalize a portion of society. To this was added an unconfirmed opinion (later rejected by medical workers) that unvaccinated people were capable of infecting vaccinated ones. Society became divided to a hitherto unseen extent, which one commentator described thus: 'The virus will subside, and the hospitals will empty, but the country will stay carved up, torn up, and disfigured by dreadful micro and macro social antipathies' (Paulius Jurkevičius 2020).

A discourse of segregation and discrimination

2021 was marked by several events that decisively shaped the course of the pandemic: the introduction of the vaccine passport in May, the end of the second quarantine at the beginning of July, the appearance of several social movements and their mass demonstrations in May, August and September, and, from the middle of September onwards, severe demands on those without a vaccine passport. The middle of September also marked the beginning of a period of segregation of the unvaccinated, a period that lasted until 5 February, when the vaccine passport was abolished. This period culminated in the barefoot mothers' protest against the vaccine passport for children and the failure of the Lithuanian Parliament's attempt at the end of the year to make vaccination compulsory for medical personnel and social workers. With the appearance of the omicron variant, which was equally dangerous to the vaccinated and unvaccinated, the pandemic situation essentially changed. The keywords for this period, in addition to those noted previously, were as follows: new COVID cases, per diem, the number of cases, due to coronavirus, people died, the numbers exceeded, infected people died, vaccines from COVID, etc.

The pandemic discourse at the beginning of 2021 did not differ from that at the end of the previous one. Those constantly supporting the Lithuanian government, the sharp-toothed commentators, continued to lash out at the enemies of vaccination. To make the discourse more effective, claims were exaggerated, and well-known words of the National Anthem were changed into their semantic opposites. Thus, instead of 'with light and truth always guiding our steps', the changed version read 'with darkness and lies always guiding our steps' (Valatka 2021a).

This tendency was most evident in attempts to create a portrait of 'modernity's enemy – the antivaxxer' according to the same principle as was used in picturing conspiracy theories. The idea was to throw everything onto the same heap. So, what are the antivaxxers like? They are homophobes, enemies of western democracies, pro-Russian sympathizers, anti-Christian pagans, sworn anti-Semites, nationalists with a special dislike for Poles, haters of businesspeople, opponents of ratifying the Istanbul Convention, beaters of their own children, haters of Landsbergis and those who, rather than blaming themselves, blame others for all the misfortunes befalling them.

Public intellectuals also spoke about the much more frequently used term science, the meaning and functions of which noticeably changed. It is this term that moved to the centre of the discord, dividing Lithuania into those who believe in science – the educated people who were vaccinated – and those who don't believe in it – the supporters of conspiracy theories who refused vaccination. After the Family March, which took place on 15 May 2021, Andrius Jakučiūnas (2021a) stated that

> the reason for the appearance and growth of a class of informal marginals lies in part with the camp of progressives themselves, who always sought to distance themselves from dissidents and used a denigrating and mocking way of speaking about them.

Nida Vasiliauskaitė and other public intellectuals also wrote about the obscurity of the phenomenon called science (Vasiliauskaitė 2021a). She analysed its popular conception, as propagated by the media, through constructions with the phrase 'scientists have proven'. Her ironic narration, tending towards sarcasm, about the banalities that so-called 'experts' discuss in news portals, ended with the following conclusion: 'science is a tool of social and political control, an institution for the shutting of mouths.'

Another feature of this period is the appearance of new genres of present-day public discourse such as satire and literary allegory, along with parodies of 'faith in science'. One of them (Jakučiūnas 2021b) depicted a situation in which all the vaccinated start growing horns. Another allegory (Vasiliauskaitė 2021c) took the reader to a medieval king's court, where the townspeople were forced to imbibe mixtures and concoctions and were seriously censored. The story mentioned 'gifts of science' and stated that the government and progressive citizens were 'going onwards in union with science'. Both allegories ironized the existing situation subtly and figuratively.

After the vaccine passport was introduced in May 2021 and the quarantine was replaced with a state of emergency at the beginning of summer, proposals to restrict or even entirely abolish individuals' constitutional rights and freedoms for the sake of the 'common good' began to be voiced ever more loudly. An influence here was the Family March, where protesters marched against the ratification of the Istanbul Convention and same-sex marriages, in addition to the vaccine passport. Their meetings poured oil onto the fire of public discourse. In addition, the Lithuanian government was the source of disquieting rumours that a new quarantine might be imposed along with additional restrictions on those without a vaccine passport. Some of these new restrictions were not approved (including closing access to public transportation to those not possessing a vaccine passport, etc.), but others came into force in the middle of September. At the same time, new voices were heard in addition to those from the previously active public intellectuals.

The old voices continued to sing the same song in much of the same key. Gintautas Mažeikis (2021a) ventured to take a study conducted in 1950 in the United States by Theodor Adorno and his colleagues on the characteristics of an authoritarian personality and apply it to the Family March participants in contemporary Lithuania – with the hope that this study would explain why the latter protest against several different things at the same time: vaccination, homosexuals and the ratification in Lithuania of the Istanbul Convention. The explanation he found was that 'the fear of infection and of homosexuality are directly interconnected'.

This line of argumentation was continued by Rimvydas Valatka (2021b). Urging people to get vaccinated, he attempted to diagnose certain opponents with 'mass suicide syndrome', and, citing examples from the practice of other nations, he made fun of the demands voiced at the meeting to reject the restrictions on rights and freedoms and urged people to make use of constitutional liberties, including the most radical one – the liberty to die free. Later, supporting the Lithuanian government's attempts to force unvaccinated people to get vaccinated, Gintautas Mažeikis (2021b) wrote about the necessity of mobilization and forced vaccination in a text that was a direct invitation to fight the antivaxxers. He was seconded by Paulius Jurkevičius (2022), who urged people 'not to waste time on antivaxxers'. Romas Sadauskas-Kvietkevičius (2022) repeated a metaphorical thought supposedly voiced by a member of the European Parliament to the effect that maintaining social contact with someone who is not vaccinated is like getting into a car driven by a drunk. Thus, the discourse that accentuated social divisions was escalated further.

However, new voices also emerged that evinced rhetoric that was without irony, sarcasm, insults or mocking. Their texts appeared in September when restrictions on unvaccinated people increased. These texts, which were not limited to the pandemic, were distinguished by their calm and matter-of-fact language, their attention more to content than to form and their greater range of topics discussed. The genres also differed: they included not only signed commentaries but also analyses, interviews and occasional speeches.

Vidas Rachlevičius wrote a sharp and frank analytic piece on the faults of Lithuanian democracy (Rachlevičius 2021a). In it, he reviewed two meetings of the Family March, one that took place in Vingis Park in May and the other near the Lithuanian Parliament in August. The reviewer called the latter a 'festival of hysteria, whipped up by a handful of commentators and influencers employing a vulgar lexicon broadcast unfiltered by the media'. In the author's opinion, the perversions of Lithuanian democracy (of which he mentions five) arise from the fact 'that loyalty to a specific government is treated as loyalty to the state itself'.

In an interview, the philosopher Alvydas Jokūbaitis (Laučius 2021) also did not approve of the government's behaviour or decision to introduce the vaccine passport.

> Concern for people's health should not step over their liberty. The pandemic only sharpened the problems of democracy. The government is accused of violating human rights, unduly restricting individual freedom, and stepping on democracy. Lithuanian political life begins to be justified by utilitarian philosophy, and the promotion of compulsory vaccination is incompatible with human dignity.

Alvydas Jokūbaitis added that 'the pandemic is not just the pandemic but has turned into a separate political phenomenon'. He was probably the first public intellectual to frankly admit that 'we do not yet understand the nature of this new development and therefore live in fear. [...] The more we do not find the right words for this new reality, the more self-confident we pretend to be'.

Attorney Ignas Vėgėlė (2021a) also criticized the government for undertaking compulsory vaccination, which he viewed as a consequence of world globalization as 'international organizations and commercial structures become the global executive government'. He claimed that 'human liberties and rights are respected only to the extent they do not violate the essential utilitarian principle of benefits and costs'. Different from other commentators on the pandemic, however, he did not raise tensions and increase antagonism but instead simply urged people to ignore the tension around the quarantine and the psychosis of the social networks and remain united.

An entirely different opinion on unity was voiced by Vidas Rachlevičius (2021b), who sought to determine the causes of diversification and the inability to communicate. In his view, public space was still a place where illusions about the president or politicians who could unify everyone were fostered, although at the same time, a very aggressive segregation of society was being carried out, leading to 'two separate Lithuanias'. According to him:

> Society is being antagonized on three main battlefields. They are COVID-19, climate change and the ideology of genderism. [...] An obvious standard and systematic method is being applied – selectivity. Those educated and believing in science do not wish to hear or see anything other, they unconditionally and enthusiastically approve of all draconian methods and restrictions. Cranking up the old record player, they pretend not to see the mass protests taking place in the Netherlands, Belgium, and Austria, and in front of Lithuania's parliament it wasn't just a shoving match between hooligans but even guns came into play. What were these all idiots and fifth columnists?

Vidas Rachlevičius concluded his commentary by saying that 'there is no possibility of reaching agreement on anything because there just is no desire to talk about it, and the verbal aggression creates a vicious circle which it is impossible to step out of'.

In a text that appeared at year's end, while pleading for unity, Ignas Vėgėlė (2021b) spoke about the 'pandemic of fear, discrimination, antagonism, humiliation, and unlawfulness' taking place against the background of the migrant and foreign policy crisis. He stated that the efficacy of COVID-19 vaccines diminishes faster than thought, there aren't any vaccines at all for the omicron variety and the problems raised in 2021 by the pandemic have merged with other, purely political, difficulties, which can be solved only by strong leadership.

Confrontational and consolidating discourse

During a meeting in 2022 in remembrance of the murderous violence unleashed by Soviet forces on 13 January 1991, protesters separated by fences from the Lithuanian Parliament drowned out some of the speakers with their whistle-cries and were therefore identified as not being Lithuanian citizens and instead denounced as members of Jedinstva (a pro-Soviet Lithuanian organization active around 1990). The Lithuanian government managed to stop the vaccination passport from coming into force before its legality began to be discussed by the Constitutional Court. The latter decided not to deliberate on the passport's legality after the government withdrew its support for it, with the option of resuming it in the future. The commemoration of 16 February 1918, the day Lithuanian independence was declared for the first time, was comparatively tranquil; in the joint crowd of both camps, one could hear the voices of both those supporting the government and those opposing it. A frequent list of keywords and key phrases from this period showed that sports events got more popular, pushing down pandemic keywords lower. However, the names of astrologers and their horoscopes retained their top positions – a sign of uncertainty prevailing in the society.

The commemorations at the beginning of 2022 of important national political events raised a new storm of discussion. It might have appeared that they passed beyond the limits of pandemic discourse, but they simply confirmed the attitudes and the social cleavage that emerged with COVID-19.

After the commemoration of 13 January, Vidas Rachlevičius (2022) declared, 'The government separated itself from the people by authoritarian fences. The question, of course, is rhetorical: can you be in the government if you do not talk with, if you sincerely hate a large portion of your country's people?' Other authors claimed that it was the so-called fifth column that had gathered in front of the Parliament and that these people had ruined the celebration because they belonged to the Jedinstva. Vidas Rachlevičius asked:

> Angry ladies and gentlemen, how many mocking sneers emanating from all possible media channels including the public broadcaster can a dissident human being quietly endure? For more than half a year Lithuania is living through a government-blessed show of hatred, and I won't mention the well-known labels, but Professor Vytautas Landsbergis, having stated that those protesting on January 13 should not be called persons of Lithuania, seemingly brought the discussion to an end.
>
> (2022)

Several days later, Landsbergis apologized on Facebook, in a very unusual way, to those he had 'injured', thereby insulting them even more with his usual irony and subtle subtexts, which can be understood and interpreted in a variety of ways. Generalizing about the political situation, Vidas Rachlevičius (2022) claimed:

> The political landscape and emotive atmosphere pushed some people toward passive resistance to this government and forced others to vent their anger in social networks or to go out on the streets and squares and whistle and shout. Hence, we have a never-before-seen social antagonism and a real Cold War. Each government gets what it deserves, it reaps what it sows.

At the beginning of the year, the event that was directly related to the management of the pandemic was the stopping of the vaccine passports coming into effect. That document was the instrument that divided Lithuanian society the most. In the public sphere, its cancellation was presented metaphorically through images of death and burial. The first to do this was the prime minister, who joked in a government meeting that when she was announcing the decision to halt the vaccination passport, she felt 'as if she were reading an obituary'. In her view, 'this tool was working, it allowed opening, not closing, perhaps it convinced one or another person to get vaccinated and protect his or her health'. In other words, she acknowledged that this was a compulsory tool for managing the pandemic that had been only provisionally discontinued and, therefore, available for reinstatement 'if the need arises'. However, the critically inclined commentators extended the metaphor and spoke of the document's burial.

In addition to examples of discourse documenting segregation at the beginning of 2022, there were examples of a consolidating discourse. In reports about the celebration of 16 February, the president was described as inviting people to extend their hand to those of another persuasion. In addition, the former chairman of Lithuania's Supreme Council, Vytautas Landsbergis (2022), stated that 'we sang out beautifully our freedom, but how do we free Lithuania's heart from the pandemic of hatred, from an indifference to everything, and even from revenge that you don't matter much?'. He warned that 'the heartless world will not survive; it will go down in the torment of fear and anger' before adding, 'what we need the least is competition among each other and internal disputes'.

Of this entire period, it can be said that the consolidating discourse that existed – to the extent it could be seen in the media – did not outweigh the confrontational one.

Brief comments on language

The pandemic discourse narrative, which contains many examples of authentic language, reveals the linguistic quality of texts on this topic. What strikes the eye the most are the changes that took place in the meaning of some words. Mokslas (science), which in Lithuanian was already an abstract noun meaning both a system of (items of) knowledge and learning, changed in its use during the pandemic with the appearance of frequently used collocations, such as *tikėti mokslu* (believe in science), *mokslo įrodyta* (science has shown), *mokslas sako* (science says) and *mokslas neatsako į klausimą* (science does not answer the question). These and other abstracts personified and humanized by metaphors of *mokslas* (science) were raised to such a level of abstractness and generalization that it made all counterarguments impossible since it remained unclear what would stand behind *mokslas* (science). As Aldous Huxley correctly remarked, 'abstract and ambiguous notions with evaluative connotations are designed with the aim to dehumanize people and to personify abstract entities' (Huxley 1936).

In addition, a metaphorized concept of *mokslas* (science) acquired a connotation of dependability and incorrigibility, with qualities of *mokslas* (science) as an object of faith or of religion, or of some kind of guarantee, mixed in. Commentators who noticed these changes remarked that in public discourse, *mokslas* (science) lost its earlier sense of intellectual activity as soon as it began to be used for propaganda purposes. The same happened with the related noun *mokslininkai* (scientists). This word tended to be used in a generalized, though not metaphorical, way. *Mokslininkai* (scientists) were mentioned without naming them personally or institutionally or specifying their science. In news portals, *mokslininkai* (scientists) were mentioned anonymously, most often in the plural, since a single *mokslininkas* (scientist) would have to be named personally. The anonymous plural reference to *mokslininkai* (scientists) usually occurred in the collocation for *mokslininkai įrodė, kad* (scientists proved that), followed by naming long-known facts or things not requiring proof (e.g. that wisdom is acquired with the passage of years, that dogs help alleviate stress, that girls mature earlier than boys, and so on). These abstract and propagandistically used words also include *ekspertai* (experts).

Two other now much more frequently used lexemes and collocations – *antivakseris* (antivaxxer) and *sąmokslo teorija* (conspiracy theory), also used primarily in the plural (*antivakseriai*) and (*sąmokslo teorijos*) – stand out with their especially denigrating connotation. *Antivakseriai* began to be applied to anyone not vaccinated against COVID-19, even if they had received shots against other diseases; whereas *sąmokslo teorijos* came to be applied to any sort of deliberation, opinion or prognosis that did not coincide with the official one, even if it later proved to be correct; for example, that unvaccinated people would be subject to stronger restrictions. In other words, connotations overcame and erased the primary meanings of words. This is a phenomenon of political language described by George Orwell, one whose semantic indefiniteness allows for the manipulation of concepts by exploiting their strong connotations. Ambiguity and lack of precision being two features of a political language, Orwell elaborated on the idea of vague or even contradictory meanings of words, stating that 'many political words are similarly abused. The word fascism has now no meaning except in so far as it signifies "something not desirable", whereas "democracy", without fail, carries positive connotation'. Moreover, Orwell highlighted that words of this kind are often used in a consciously dishonest way (Orwell 1946). Even though, compared to *mokslas* (science) and *mokslininkai* (scientists), the connotations of *antivakseris* and *sąmokslo teorija* are opposite in intent, what is common to them is overgeneralization and ambiguity.

The phrase 'social distance', having become another keyword of the COVID-19 discourse, is also not used in its usual sense. In the context of the pandemic, it meant the physical distance which must be kept rather than the social distance between different social classes or people having nothing in common except that in some sense they happen to be near to one another. The requirement to observe a social, but not a physical, distance, if we understand this phrase correctly, is a case of verbal aggression. The Global Initiative on Psychiatry (Robert van Voren 2020, 2022) suggested that social distance be changed to the more accurate term physical/space distance, which is what is really needed during a pandemic, whereas social distance implies unnecessary alienation.

One more example of distorted semantics is *galimybių pasas* (a Lithuanian phrase for vaccine passport), initially called *žaliasis pasas* (green passport) through analogy with traffic light colours. In English, this document was called a QR code or immunity pass without any evaluative connotations. Now *galimybių pasas* is a typical euphemism in political language as discussed by George Orwell. It is intended to cover up the unpleasant sides of a phenomenon of reality and highlight the brighter ones. Both words of the Lithuanian term were criticized for different reasons. The first word *galimybių* because of its euphemistic sense, as opposed to its announced meaning, since for more than half of inhabitants, it took away rather than added possibilities, thus making it an obvious instance of segregation or of so-called epidemic racism. The second word *pasas* because a notice of health is labelled in such a way that it is raised to the level of the most important state document, a passport showing its bearer to be a citizen.

A distinctive part of the pandemic lexicon was constituted by neologisms, mostly formed by blending. Thus, we got *plandemija* from *planuota pandemija* (planned pandemia); *infodemija* from *informacijos pandemija* (information pandemia); *kovidiotai* from *kovido idiotai* (COVID idiots); *chamentarai* from *chamiški komentarai* (asshole comments); *bufonautai* from *boo šaukiantys ufonautai* (booing UFOs); *bukalaurai* from *buki bakalaurai* (bungling bachelors); *bobausybė* from *bobų vyriausybė* (broads' government), and so on. Most of these neologisms have a negative connotation; they are insulting, and they amplify the irritation of pandemic communication. Sometimes, the negative connotation is orthographic, as when, wishing to diminish someone, a person's surname is written with a small first letter, especially when a proper noun coincides with a common noun. For example, *vėgėlė* is both an attorney's surname and the name of a fish.

Expressions much more commonly used include those associated not so much with the pandemic directly, but with the function of the discourse about it. These are hyperbolized expressions, such as *užsikrėtimų protrūkis* (breakout of infections), *pavojaus sirenos* (sirens of danger), *mirčių rekordas* (record deaths), *pacientų antplūdis* (flood of patients), *ruoštis blogiausiam* (to prepare for the worst), *pandemija siautėja* (the pandemic is raging), *didžiausias atvejų prieaugis* (the biggest increase in cases), *rekordiškai daug naujų atvejų* (a record number of new cases).

Military terms and metaphors also increased in the frequency of their use. These deserve more attention because many linguists, especially the cognitivists, recognize the effect that metaphors have on language users, in particular, their power. That power manifests itself not only in understanding and experiencing reality, but also in accepting the appropriateness of war:

> We clearly recognize the power of language. Nevertheless, we use a great deal of violent language in ordinary everyday speech quite oblivious of the way in which we are constructing our language to glorify war and violence and, in that way, make such violence appear appropriate even acceptable when it appears in reality.
> (Hardman 2002)

He claims that the war metaphor plants seeds of violence. A similar evaluation of the war metaphor comes from Lakoff and Frisch (2006) in the context of the events of 9/11: 'the war metaphor created a new reality that reinforced the metaphor.' The latter and the language of war in general greatly reduced opportunities to look for solutions other than confrontation: 'Locked in the language of war, it's impossible to find another way out' (Katz 2004). This is specifically addressed by the media, which tends to be biased in choosing a specific vocabulary for the language of war. Media in post-Soviet countries is notorious for the overuse of war metaphors (Marcinkevičienė 2012).

The words and phrases mentioned here, along with their semantics, involve the special lexicon of the pandemic. The pandemic syntax shows a predilection for frequent rhetorical questions, especially in the commentaries, and for a dictatorial tone in the government's information messages 'from now on it will be like this' (Aleksandravičius 2021).

Looking at the issue more broadly, on a textual level, we would notice that in the evaluative genres, especially the commentaries, irony and sarcasm predominate. Entire texts are written ironically, and for the irony to not be so biting, the persons at whom it is directed are referred to indirectly, for example, the creator of luxury goods, the first philosopher of the second Lithuania, Mister Global and the managers of the pandemic. This is done to encrypt the persons mentioned but not so radically that this bubble's readers would not be able to determine who was being talked about, and the authors could avoid accusations that they were insulting someone. This is a distinguishing feature of certain pandemic texts, an element of argot that makes the language vague or ambiguous and sometimes hard to decipher.

The language of pandemic discourse and its effect on society are best described by a quotation from George Orwell. In his seminal essay 'Politics and the English language' (1946), in which he expands on the links between language and thought, he writes: 'But if thought corrupts language, language can also corrupt thought'. He believes that the political chaos that is connected to the decay of language can be diminished 'by starting at the verbal end' and that human language can be shaped for our own purposes. He argues that this shaping should include awareness and conscious refusal of certain bad features of language.

Concluding remarks and an epilogue

The role of language and the impact of words on our health and well-being has always been big; however, during the pandemic, it became even bigger since mediated communication deprived us of its non-verbal part (gestures, body language) that conveyed meaning and speaker's intension alongside with language. Meanwhile, public communication, media in particular, became much more important in everyday life as news outlets had a direct influence on lives and everyday activities. News portals increased their readership and naturally their influence on society.

The research on public media discourse revealed its prevailing functions during COVID-19, i.e. to express irritation and to cause intimidation with a focus on dissatisfaction with the situation, feelings of insecurity and societal problems caused by COVID-19. Besides, most media highlighted distrust, miscommunication and the atmosphere of fear predominantly presented in dramatic and hyperbolized expressions. Combined with the contents of threatening news the negativism of expression, and military rhetorics that usually pop up in times of crises as well as in authoritarian regimes, it caused a bipolar way of thinking that infected social relations. People were trapped by the confrontational pattern of thought, and with the help of linguistic expressions two opposing camps were formed, and two sides of barricades were constructed. Their opinions were expressed in the most radical forms of linguistic aggression ranging from angry irritation to bullying or even virtual violence. It is hard to say whether the discoursal mechanisms mentioned above are just outcomes of societal crises or whether they become more expressed and more visible during crises. In any case, they make crises even worse and more dangerous. One can only wonder what our society would have been like now if the pandemic discourse had taken on a different type of verbal expression.

The pandemic discourse ended as abruptly as it started, with the war in Ukraine taking over the news portals. A year after its end, the topic of COVID-19 appeared mostly in short and emotionally neutral news reports. Nevertheless, the topics of experiences of the pandemic and the fate of democracy did not disappear altogether, they found their reflections in a range of genres in fiction (from short stories to dystopian novels) and even in poetry. Thus, in a different discourse, more distant from everyday reality, abstract and elevated, philosophically grounded, and devoid of social confrontation. What remained in post-COVID media discourse was its inclination to intimidate its readers and continue with a bipolar approach using any other topics at hand for that aim.

REFERENCES

Aleknavičė, Karolina (2021), 'Gintautas Mažeikis apie tai, kodėl tikime sąmokslo teorijomis ir kaip su jomis kovoti: vos tik uždrausi, iškart suvešės', *15min.lt*, 12 February, https://www.15min.lt/naujiena/aktualu/lietuva/g-mazeikis-apie-tai-kodel-tikime-samokslo-teorijomis-ir-kaip-su-jomis-kovoti-vos-tik-uzdrausi-iskart-isveses-56-1452788. Accessed 20 April 2023.

Aleksandravičius, Egidijus (2021), 'Lex ex Deo', *LRT.lt*, 29 December, https://www.lrt.lt/naujienos/nuomones/3/1571681/egidijus-aleksandravicius-lex-ex-deo. Accessed 20 April 2023.

Fairclough, Norman (1995), *Critical Discourse Analysis*, London: Longman.

Hardman, M. J. (2002), 'Language and war', *First Published on International Humanist News February 2002*, https://humanists.international/news/. Accessed 16 August 2010.

Huxley, Aldous (1936), *Words and Behaviour*, pp. 1265–79, https://www.sevanoland.com/uploads/1/1/8/0/118081022/words_and_behavior.pdf. Accessed 20 April 2023.

Jakučiūnas, Andrius (2020), 'Mėšlakalbiai prie "bybianosius". Apmaudžios lygiosios', *15min.lt*, 5 November, https://www.15min.lt/kultura/naujiena/asmenybe/andrius-jakuciunas-meslakalbiai-pries-bybianosius-apmaudzios-lygiosios-285-1402348. Accessed 20 April 2023.

Jakučiūnas, Andrius (2021a), 'Apie šešis milijardus homofobų ir burtažodį "mokslas"', *15min.lt*, 11 June, https://www.15min.lt/kultura/naujiena/asmenybe/andrius-jakuciunas-apie-sesis-milijardus-homofobu-ir-burtazodi-mokslas-285-1518906. Accessed 20 April 2023.

Jakučiūnas, Andrius (2021b), 'O kas, jei nuo skiepų išdygtų ragai?' *15min.lt*, 28 August, https://www.15min.lt/kultura/naujiena/asmenybe/andrius-jakuciunas-o-kas-jei-nuo-skiepu-isdygtu-ragai-285-1556066. Accessed 20 April 2023.

Jurkevičius, Paulius (2020), 'Prezidente, o jūs paskui mus sutaikysite?' *Delfi.lt*, 12 December, https://www.delfi.lt/news/ringas/lit/paulius-jurkevicius-prezidente-o-jus-paskui-mus-sutaikysite.d?id=85973611. Accessed 20 April 2023.

Jurkevičius, Paulius (2022), 'Šeštoji, itališka pavara: nesiterlioti su antivakseriais', *Delfi.lt*, 15 January, https://www.delfi.lt/news/ringas/lit/paulius-jurkevicius-sestoji-italiska-pavara-nesiterlioti-su-antivakseriais.d?id=89202479. Accessed 20 April 2023.

Kalinauskaitė, Danguolė and Aleksandravičiūtė-Šviažienė, Austė (2020), 'Headlines in the context of the pandemic: The communication of irritation', *Deeds and Days*, 74, pp. 181–99. https://doi.org/10.7220/2335-8769.74.9.

Katz, Eliot (2004), 'Unlocking the language room of war', *First Published on September 7, 2004 by CommonDreams.org*, https://www.eliotkatzpoetry.com/unlocking-the-language-room-of-war/. Accessed 20 April 2023.

Lakoff, George and Frish, Evan (2006), 'Five years after 9/11: Drop the war metaphor', *First Published on September 11, 2006 by CommonDreams.org*, https://www.huffpost.com/entry/five-years-after-911-drop_b_29181. Accessed 20 April 2023.

Landsbergis, Vytautas (2022), 'Mums mažiausiai reikia tarpusavio varžybų ir vidaus peštynių', *Verslo žinios.lt*, 16 February, https://www.vz.lt/verslo-aplinka/2022/02/16/v-landsbergis-mums-maziausiai-reikia-tarpusavio-varzybu-ir-vidaus-pestyniu. Accessed 20 April 2023.

Laučius, Vladimiras (2021), 'Alvydas Jokubaitis: negalima reikalauti atsakomybės iš vergo', *Delfi.lt*, 17 September, https://www.delfi.lt/news/daily/lithuania/alvydas-jokubaitis-negalima-reikalauti-atsakomybes-is-vergo.d?id=88190917. Accessed 20 April 2023.

Marcinkevičienė, Rūta (2012), 'A dangerous language', in K. Gouliamos and Ch. Kassimeris (eds), *The Marketing of War in the Age of Neo-Militarism*, New York and London: Routledge, pp. 23–41.

Mažeikis, Gintautas (2020a), 'Karūnos virusas ir A.Camus "Maras"', *VDU.lt*, 16 March, https://www.vdu.lt/lt/gintautas-mazeikis-karunos-virusas-ir-a-camus-maras/. Accessed 20 April 2023.

Mažeikis, Gintautas (2020b) 'Sienų ir ribų sugrįžimas', *15min.lt*, 9 April, https://www.15min.lt/naujiena/aktualu/komentarai/gintautas-mazeikis-sienu-ir-ribu-sugrizimas-500-1302086. Accessed 20 April 2023.

Mažeikis, Gintautas (2021a), 'Skiepai, homofobija ir autoritarizmas', *LRT.lt*. 13 September, https://www.lrt.lt/naujienos/nuomones/3/1495293/gintautas-mazeikis-skiepai-homofobija-ir-autoritarizmas. Accessed 20 April 2023.

Mažeikis, Gintautas (2021b), 'Apie mobilizacijos ir prievartos skiepytis būtinybę', *LRT.lt*, 3 November, https://www.lrt.lt/naujienos/nuomones/3/1533397/gintautas-mazeikis-apie-mobilizacijos-ir-prievartos-skiepytis-butinybe. Accessed 20 April 2023.

Orwell, George (1946), 'Politics and the English language', https://www.orwellfoundation.com/the-orwell-foundation/orwell/essays-and-other-works/politics-and-the-english-language/. Accessed 20 April 2023.

Rachlevičius, Vidas (2021a), 'Lietuviškoji demokratija: teoriškai – arklys, praktiškai – neatsikelia', *Delfi.lt*, 2 September, https://www.delfi.lt/news/ringas/lit/vidas-rachlevicius-lietuviskoji-demokratija-teoriskai-arklys-praktiskai-neatsikelia.d?id=88075489. Accessed 20 April 2023.

Rachlevičius, Vidas (2021b), 'Vieninga tauta – naivi iliuzija. Mes niekada nebesusikalbėsime', *Delfi.lt*, 13 December, https://www.delfi.lt/news/ringas/lit/vidas-rachlevicius-vieninga-tauta-naivi-iliuzija-mes-niekada-nebesusikalbesime.d?id=88903211. Accessed 20 April 2023.

Rachlevičius, Vidas (2022), 'Ponios ir ponai, ar ne laikas prilaikyti arklius?' *Delfi.lt*, 18 January, https://www.delfi.lt/news/ringas/lit/vidas-rachlevicius-ponios-ir-ponai-ar-ne-laikas-prilaikyti-arklius.d?id=89229533. Accessed 20 April 2023.

Sadauskas-Kvietkevičius, Romas (2022), 'Aš tai kitaip pandemiją valdyčiau', *Delfi.lt*, 29 January, https://m.delfi.lt/ringas/article.php?id=89319177. Accessed 20 April 2023.

Valatka, Rimvydas (2020), 'Jie nesiskiepys. 23rk ą jūs jiiems padarysit?' *Delfi.lt*, 13 December, https://www.delfi.lt/news/ringas/lit/rimvydas-valatka-jie-nesiskiepys-ir-ka-jus-jiems-padarysit.d?id=85987915. Accessed 20 April 2023.

Valatka, Rimvydas (2021a), 'Rauna stogus. 8 patarimai vyriausybei', *Delfi.lt*, 7 February.

Valatka, Rimvydas (2021b), 'Pilėnų sindromas', *Delfi.lt*, 17 October, https://www.delfi.lt/news/ringas/lit/rimvydas-valatka-pilenu-sindromas.d?id=88447635. Accessed 20 April 2023.

Van Voren, Robert (2020), 'Kartu per atstumą', 6 May, https://www.youtube.com/watch?v=2yt-G787aazI. Accessed 20 April 2023.

Van Voren, Robert (2022), 'Society and the individual: from Soviet psychiatric terror to COVID-19', *Deeds and Days*, 77, pp. 143–59, https://doi.org/10.7220/2335-8769.77.8.

Vasiliauskaitė, Nida (2020a), 'Apie sąmokslus ir teorijas', *Delfi.lt*, 21 April, https://www.delfi.lt/news/ringas/lit/nida-vasiliauskaite-apie-samokslus-ir-teorijas.d?id=84086613. Accessed 20 April 2023.

Vasiliauskaitė, Nida (2020b), 'Apie konspiratorių medžioklę', *Delfi.lt*, 30 November, https://www.delfi.lt/news/ringas/lit/nida-vasiliauskaite-apie-konspiratoriu-medziokle.d?id=85804161. Accessed 20 April 2023.

Vasiliauskaitė, Nida (2021a), 'Mokslas, arba naujasis obskurantizmas', *Delfi.lt*, 25 February, https://www.delfi.lt/news/ringas/lit/nida-vasiliauskaite-mokslas-arba-naujasis-obskurantizmas.d?id=86533317. Accessed 20 April 2023.

Vasiliauskaitė, Nida (2021b), 'Apie "mitų" griovėjus', *Delfi.lt*, 17 March, https://www.delfi.lt/news/ringas/lit/nida-vasiliauskaite-apie-mitu-griovejus.d?id=86708897. Accessed 20 April 2023.

Vasiliauskaitė, Nida (2021c), 'Karantino istorijos', *Delfi.lt*, 19 April, https://www.delfi.lt/news/ringas/lit/nida-vasiliauskaite-karantino-istorijos.d?id=86949323. Accessed 20 April 2023.

Vėgėlė, Ignas (2021a), 'Visa I.Vėgėlės kalba apie skiepijimą. Įvertinkite patys', *15min.lt*, 23 August, https://www.15min.lt/naujiena/aktualu/nuomones/visa-i-vegeles-kalba-apie-skiepijima-ivertinkite-patys-18-1553550. Accessed 20 April 2023.

Vėgėlė, Ignas (2021b), 'Iracionalios politikos kakofonija. Metas prezidento lyderystei', *Delfi.lt*, 28 December, https://www.delfi.lt/news/ringas/lit/ignas-vegele-iracionalios-politikos-kakofonija-metas-prezidento-lyderystei.d?id=89059641. Accessed 20 April 2023.

Wodak, Ruth and Meyer, Michael (2001), *Methods of Critical Discourse Analysis*, Thousand Oaks, CA: Sage Publications.

CREATIVE RESPONSES
TO PLAGUE

11

Nights of Crises and Resistance: (En)countering the Politics of Disease and Death in *Bacurau* (2019)

Sara Brandellero

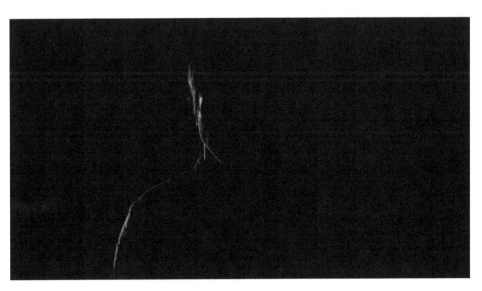

FIGURE 11.1: Frame grab from *Bacurau*, 2019. Courtesy of Kleber Mendonça Filho, at Cinemascopio.

This chapter discusses representations of night-time and darkness in the acclaimed 2019 feature film *Bacurau* by Brazilian directors Kleber Mendonça Filho and Juliano Dornelles. It considers the role played by spaces filmed under the cover of darkness in the film's representation of social crises in public health provision and wellbeing. This chapter draws on Williams' (2008) spatialized conceptualization of the night, understood as comprising the part of the 24-hour cycle that is commonly associated with life after dark. Williams argues that dimensions of time and space cannot be uncoupled and defends the conceptualization of 'night spaces' as distinctive from daytime spatialities. Following Williams, this chapter conceives of night spaces as socially mediated and related to 'processes of territorialization': social forms of imposition or attempts by authorities to impose order on the interactions between people and on the non-human world (Williams 2008: 517).

In this discussion of the nocturnal time–space, this chapter will draw on the image of the *terreiro*, a Portuguese word with meanings ranging from 'yard' to 'square', and which is strongly associated with spaces of African Brazilian cultural practices and resistance that are often played out at night and which seem to resonate in the filmic configurations of Bacurau.

In line with these considerations, this chapter contends that the nocturnal time–space underpins the film's imaginative storytelling of historic, deep-rooted social inequality and injustice, envisaging the embattled small Brazilian town of Bacurau as an enclave of community resilience and resistance against state-sponsored political, technological, economic and health warfare. The town's racially and gender diverse community holds out in one of Brazil's most impoverished regions in the face of relentless 'forms of subjugating life to the power of death', as Mbembe (2019: 92) conceptualizes necropolitical practices.

The film's title invites a closer analysis of the significance of the night, which has been overlooked in earlier critical appraisals. As will be discussed in detail below, the fictional town of Bacurau takes its name from a bird of prey that lives in the wild and comes out at night. Since a number of the film's most stunning sequences are set at night, this chapter will investigate how the nocturnal time–space, in its symbolic and material representations, contributes to the film's engagement with questions of social justice that have health and wellbeing at their core. As will be discussed in the sections that follow, the film invites us to enter into the night as a territory occupied by a diverse community marginalized by lopsided power structures.

Thus, this study builds on previous critical discussions of *Bacurau* in addressing the significance of the night, which has remained something of a blind spot in earlier readings. Critics have commented on the film's stunning mix of cinematic genres and its engagement with Brazil's political cinematic tradition (e.g. Bentes 2019; Ikeda 2020), also in light of the COVID-19 pandemic (Fischer 2021). Generally considered a film that celebrates popular resistance, it has nonetheless, for some critics, proved controversial in what some see as its mainstream spectacularizing of violence and skewed representation of racial and gender diversity, in which representations of lesbian identities and desires, for example, end up being tokenistic. Also controversial is its ambiguous treatment of Brazil's history of racial discrimination, demonstrated by pitting the town of Bacurau against a bunch of demonized foreign mercenaries who are defenders of a white supremacist ideology and bent on annihilating the town's population of colour (e.g. Brandão and de Lira 2020; Ferreira and Nafafé 2021; Mittelman 2022). Mindful of some of the ambiguities revealed in *Bacurau*'s fictionalization of crisis and resistance, this analysis contends that the film presents an imperfect outcome in a long history dominated by politics that privileges death over life, a solution for which has yet to materialize.

In the cinematic visualization of the town's resistance, the directors' choice of location and their use of nocturnal settings draw on a rich web of experiences and symbolic connotations that have coalesced around the idea of night. Dunn and Edensor (2020: 1) remind us that 'darkness is multiple, situational, contested'. It triggers a range of associations that link the night with danger, social disorder and criminality, and, conversely, positive perceptions of the nocturnal, in which darkness, for example, affords important opportunities for resistance against oppressive systems of power (e.g. Lefebvre 1974; Chazkel 2017; Palmer 2000). Building on these complex associations, the film's engagement with social and political concerns that address questions of inequality and discrimination gained added resonance in light of the COVID-19 pandemic, especially for the Brazilian case in light of the disastrous extreme right-wing Bolsonaro government (2018–22) that was in power through that time. Indeed, *Bacurau* poignantly illustrates the prescience of the arts and artistic imaginative storytelling in instigating, galvanizing and even anticipating public debates on community justice and wellbeing.

Made in pre-pandemic times, the film is eerily resonant with the plight of millions of people affected by COVID-19 restrictions, and it envisions drastic solutions from below that have health equity at the heart of social justice and are mindful of a history of colonial, gender and racial violence. *Bacurau* does so by revealing a history of social neglect in Brazil, of which the management of the pandemic would prove a new manifestation. By adopting a historical and postcolonial perspective, *Bacurau* invites a more privileged audience from the Global North to reframe their recent experience of the health crisis against a global imbalance in wealth and healthcare justice.

Film context

Released to national and international acclaim in 2019 and winning the Jury Prize at Cannes that same year, this hybrid Sci-Fi-cum-Western-Horror feature has garnered public and critical endorsement and generated a substantial amount of controversy, with its provocative use of film genre to articulate a social and political critique of contemporary Brazil. The film's production itself represented an act of resistance vis-à-vis the attack that Brazilian cinema and the arts and culture industries more broadly have come under in the country's recent administrations (Backstein 2020) following the parliamentary coup that removed left-wing President Dilma Rousseff in 2016 and ultimately paved the way for the election of far-right President Bolsonaro (2018–22).

The film's title refers to the name of the small town in which it is set, and notably, it was also used as the title for the film's international release, drawing attention to the significance of the name, the meaning of which is not widely known, even in Brazil itself. *Bacurau* translates as 'nighthawk' in English, and we learn early on in the film from one of the town's inhabitants that the word refers to a wild bird of prey that comes out at night. In the north-east region of Brazil, where the action takes place, the word is also used to designate the last night bus, a means of transport associated with the most impoverished sections of society, especially night workers. This adds to the constellation of associations of *Bacurau* with Brazil's traditionally overlooked populations and purposefully embeds the narrative in a specific cultural/national context, instigating connections with the plight of marginalized spaces and communities in pandemic times.

Director Mendonça Filho's acclaimed earlier feature films indicated his commitment to politically and socially engaged cinematic production. *Neighbouring Sounds* (2012) and *Aquarius* (2016), both set in the north-eastern city of Recife, take on issues of social inequality and injustice in urban Brazil and highlight their roots in the country's history as a colonial, rural, slave-based economy and patriarchal societal structures. The films address questions of racial, class and gender discrimination, as well as the inequality that has persisted in a country where social and political structures of privilege have remained largely untouched since colonial times. If, in both of these films, the urban context reveals how a history of inequality seeps into the present, often manifested in overt or simmering urban violence, in *Bacurau*, it is a rural setting that is in focus alongside the impact of fossilized power structures on communities that lie at the margin of a predominantly urban society.

A number of the film's key sequences take place after dark. When the town suddenly and mysteriously vanishes from the maps because their communication systems have been sabotaged by the foreign group contracted by the mayor to exterminate the locals, it becomes a poignant metaphor for the inhabitants' social and (geo)political invisibility, which is replicated in later scenes when they gather to articulate their resistance under the cover of darkness. The image included at the top of this chapter captures one moment of the night scenes in which the foreign contracted killers spread terror in the town. The image shows the barely distinguishable headshot of Joshua (Brian Townes), as he murders one of the unsuspecting town's young children who are out playing at night. The image conjures the sense of invisible danger and dystopia facing the small rural community and is a snapshot of the film's exploration of nocturnal aesthetics to channel the terror to which the people are subjected.

In the dystopian future that the film imagines, we learn early on that medical supplies and medical care are scarce and that routine vaccine supplies are withheld. Instead, the local population is plied with out-of-date mood-numbing pills. To counter this, care is organized through community solidarity, and inhabitants rely on a locally produced plant-based hallucinogenic pill that is meant to expand the mind. The village doctor, Domingas (Sônia Braga), works with the limited means at her disposal and educates the population to steer clear of the out-of-date medicines that are periodically dumped onto the townspeople by the local politician Tony Júnior (Thardelly Lima). In a stunning performance by Braga, an icon of Brazilian cinema, the character of Domingas becomes one of the key figures of the revolt that will eventually unfold as the village of Bacurau reacts to an orchestrated attack waged against its people for resisting a perverse necropolitical system.

To compound this health crisis context, shots of a derelict school building indicate the authorities' inadequate investment in education, and we also learn that the local politician is blocking the town's water supply, leaving the inhabitants of Bacurau at the mercy of deliveries from water trucks. We later discover that Tony Jr is colluding with a group of foreign, mostly North American, trigger-happy gunmen and women led by Michael (masterfully played by Udo Kier), who is tasked with killing the village population. The goal is to allow the political elite to gain full control of the distribution channels of the natural water supplies, capitalizing on the lucrative bottled water industry. Brazil's north-eastern region has been plagued by a history of droughts, which, coupled with the region's bloody history of unequal land ownership and violence against disenfranchised land labourers, makes the film's attention to the conflict over water access all the more poignant. Indeed, the prominence of the theme of water supply in the film is one of the narrative features through which the film contextualizes the current health crisis in the region within a history of neglect and (neo)colonial extractivist economies.

Images of coffins lying on the roadside and lined up in the village square allude to the state's failure to provide care and the necropolitics on which it thrives – putting profit and private interests over community wellbeing. Building on a tradition of political cinema in Brazil and Latin America more broadly, the film comments on the entanglement of a history of class, racial and gender violence, exploitative economic models and a glorification of guns and violence, of which the lack of adequate healthcare is one ramification. This imagined future order of things, which the village of Bacurau attempts to oppose, resonated with audiences witnessing Bolsonaro's Trump-inspired flippant response to the pandemic.

Questioned by a journalist about the rising death toll in April 2020, Bolsonaro gave one of his usually dismissive responses, stating, 'I'm not a gravedigger, OK?' (Gomes 2020).[1] The consequence of his disregard for public health and his dismissiveness of COVID-19 measures, in favour of sheer economic interests, would be Brazil recording the second-highest COVID-19 official death toll in the world, with close to 700,000 deaths recorded by December 2022 (WHO).

As Conde (2020) reminds us, COVID-19 was introduced to Brazil by the jet-setting elite, but the disease disproportionately affected the poorest, mostly black and indigenous, populations in the country. Historically, these groups would be most likely to live in overcrowded communities with little or no infrastructure, would have limited access to adequate medical care and would not have the luxury of being able to work from home or self-isolate. In sum, the pandemic highlighted systemic inequalities that were entrenched along race and class fault lines.

Set in a dystopian future, 'a few years from now' as the opening credits tell us, the film's shots of the lined-up coffins donated to the town's population by the corrupt Tony Jr in a cynical gesture of goodwill could not fail to remind audiences of the shocking images of mass graves that flashed across Brazil's television screens as the tragedy of the mishandled COVID-19 pandemic took hold of the country. At the same time, the gruesome gun violence that escalates as the film's narrative action unfolds, in which killing sprees are played out in a kind of videogame aesthetic (as Ferreira and Nafafé (2021) also noted), alludes to the Bolsonaro government's trivialization of gun violence and endorsement of mass firearm ownership. Describing *Bacurau* as a 'visionary and violent' film revolving around what she terms (following Sayak Valencia) the gruesome reality of 'capitalist gore', Brazilian critic Bentes defines it as 'possibly the most important contemporary film on the dystopian Brazil of the Bolsonaro era' (Bentes 2019: n.pag.).

That said, the film frames the current impasse from a historical perspective, an intention that the directors themselves acknowledged when they claimed that *Bacurau* aimed to capture some of Brazil's chronic social issues (Mendonça Filho 2019). Along similar lines, the well-known drag artist and actor Silvero Pereira, who plays Lunga, the queer rebel leader who emerges from his gang hideout on the edge of town to defend Bacurau, stated that the film did not necessarily represent the Bolsonaro government, but that 'it's about the government we've always had' (in Rubinstein 2020). At the same time, he acknowledged the advancements in LGBTQIA+ rights, specifically during Brazil's earlier progressive Lula and Rousseff governments, and identified *Bacurau* as a metaphor for the preservation of hard-won rights, as embodied in his own stunning lead role as the gender-fluid rebel character of Lunga. Turning the geographical place name into a verb of political resistance, Pereira highlighted that the need to address social inequalities for traditionally marginalized groups while holding on to recent progress remains: 'If necessary, we will *bacurize* not to lose the rights that we have achieved' (Pereira cited in Rubinstein 2020).

Mindful of this historical context, *Bacurau* poignantly treats the community as an organic whole, a common body whose inhabitants do not appear as mere 'extras' in the narrative, but as constituents of what Rubinstein defined as a 'living, breathing organism' (Rubinstein 2020; feature also mentioned by Mendonça Filho during Q&A, see recording Film at Lincoln Centre 2020).

The town's museum, a source of great pride for the local population, is repeatedly referenced by various characters and features as one of the key locations in the film's violent dénouement. Pieces on display in the museum refer to the region's history of *cangaço*, a form of rural banditry that dominated the area in the nineteenth and early part of the twentieth century. The camera pauses on newspaper cuttings of articles referring to *cangaceiros* (bandits) in their characteristic leather outfits and semi-circle-shaped hats, mapping a history of conflict between the forces of law and order and the rural gangs. They are problematic characters due to their original status as a kind of militia recruited by the rich landowners in the region and the Robin Hood status they often erroneously acquired in popular lore, thanks to their own humble origins. Such ambiguity is maintained in the ensuing drama; as violence and revenge dominate, the people of Bacurau take justice into their own hands and the final outcome points to the perpetuation of unresolved conflicts.

Night visions

The film opens with a Star Wars-inspired sequence of shots from outer space consisting of long shots of planet Earth that capture the planet surrounded by darkness. As if on board an alien spaceship, the camera takes us gradually closer to the blue planet, heading towards the surface of the Earth and eventually reaching the ground level, focusing on a moving water delivery truck travelling in Brazil's rural semi-arid outback that is heading to the location of Bacurau, which is 17 km away. This initial sequence, immersed as it is in the darkness of outer space, serves to introduce the leitmotif of the nocturnal world that will provide one of the narrative threads of the film, also connecting the plight of the previously inconspicuous town of Bacurau – a mere speck on the surface of the Earth – with a universal call for social justice.

The sequence is accompanied by the well-known sound of Brazilian songwriter Caetano Veloso's 1968 composition '*Objeto não identificado*' [Unidentified Object] in a version interpreted by his contemporary and celebrated singer Gal Costa. Representative of the trailblazing Tropicalia movement in Brazil of the late 1960s and 1970s, the song mixes electronic sounds with more traditional melodic instrumental music, exemplifying the movement's drive to update traditional Brazilian popular music by incorporating electronic instruments and influences from British and American rock music traditions.

Mattos (2019) reminds us that Tropicalia, with its iconoclastic aesthetics, was one of the artistic movements to oppose the military dictatorship that took over Brazil in 1964 and that would last until the return to democracy in 1985. This political subtext to the opening musical commentary on the film provides an early link to *Bacurau*'s political engagement. Moreover, the song's innovative mix of traditional sounds and novel, psychedelic rock-inspired arrangements indicate the film's reframing of the semi-arid, impoverished landscapes of north-east Brazil with which Brazilian cinema audiences would be familiar. In this reframing of this rural setting, the film presents an updated vision of the region, showing the persistence of poverty and social neglect alongside the widespread use of modern technology (tablets, mobile phones, etc.).

Two sequences in the film are, I argue, especially significant in the film's characterization of Bacurau as a space of resistance against oppression in this context, and both are set after nightfall. In the first, the local population gathers in the town's square to inspect the goods left by Tony Jr in his latest visit to the town as he seeks to garner votes in the forthcoming local elections. As the people congregate outside the museum building, Domingas warns them against taking home the medical supplies dumped on the town – all of which are out of date. The situation is even more serious, given that the supplies consist of a mood-numbing medication meant only for use with a medical prescription, the liberal distribution of which is creating an epidemic of medication dependency. As an alternative, the townspeople are reminded of their own production of psychotropic substances, which will eventually prove instrumental in aiding their action during the violent armed resistance that follows.

This scene serves to characterize the town's public space at night as an important reference for community building, regrouping and support. The extended night sequence that follows this, after the town has come under direct attack from the trigger-happy mercenary foreign gang, underscores the correlation between the night and the marginalized people's social invisibility. It also emerges as a metaphor for their deploying of this same invisibility to their advantage in the guerrilla-like warfare that ensues against the foreign invaders.

In this extended night-time sequence, the townspeople plan their warfare strategy alongside Lunga and his henchmen, who have joined to support the town's struggle. The night setting and dramatic use of chiaroscuro that the natural cover of darkness facilitates adds to the tension that builds in this mix of western and Sci-Fi genres. In the dystopian future that the film imagines in this small-town rural setting, the night-time scenario is deployed with a tongue-in-cheek nod to the Sci-Fi visual vocabulary that is generally urban-based. The townspeople cut through the pitch-black darkness of the town's streets, where the electricity has been cut off by the contract killers, in collusion with the mayor, in order to quickly subdue any local resistance. Several shots that show groups of townsfolk heading into the darkness capture them head-on. This has the effect of blinding the audience (and any potential attacker), thanks to the headlights being pointed directly at them, while at the same time making the organized mob of the Bacurau people invisible to their enemy against the darkness behind them.

The film's directors revealed that their chosen location for filming Bacurau is, in reality, the remnants of what is known in Brazil as a *quilombo*, a word designating a community originating from runaway enslaved people, usually located in the country's remote interior. A reference to Brazil's resistance to acknowledging its history of slavery is poignantly recalled in the night scene, as the camera dwells on a group of people practising *capoeira* accompanied by chanting and traditional drumbeats. A martial art originally developed by enslaved people and disguised as dance to avoid prohibition, *capoeira* continues to be associated with cultural practices of racial resistance. As the drumbeats are replaced with the musical commentary of John Carpenter's eerily futuristic electronic composition 'Night', the scene underscores the continuity between the struggles of the past and the unresolved injustices of the present.

As part of recent research into night spaces connected to migrant cultural practices of resistance, I interviewed the co-founder of the Dutch-Brazilian theatre group Munganga in Amsterdam at the height of the first lockdown in the summer of 2020, when no entertainment venues were open. In my conversation with actor, director, cultural producer and activist Carlos Lagoeiro, he described what the night meant to him. As a cultural producer of an independent, progressive space promoting a cultural programme of inclusion and intercultural exchange, his response was poignant. Lagoeiro spoke of the night by using the Portuguese word *terreiro*: He said: 'the night is a *terreiro*, as Munganga becomes a place of encounter and exchange between artists and the public' (Interview 30 June 2020). The Portuguese word *terreiro* literally translates into English as 'yard' but carries multiple and hybrid meanings that also conflate different temporalities, including an association with the African Brazilian history of cultural resistance. Indeed, *terreiro* can relate to a town square, to bare earth, crop cultivation, popular festivals, rituals and worship, as well as open-air spaces of labour, and is commonly associated with African Brazilian religious practices, which are mostly carried out at night and which have come under increasing violent attacks under Bolsonaro's extreme right-wing government. Thus, the image of the '*terreiro*' through which the night was imagined conjured up the experience of migrant night-time cultures as both a time and space that connect to a history of resistance, heritage, regeneration, communal wellbeing and care. Its significance for migrant and diasporic communities' wellbeing was thrown into greater relief once government measures, fear of disease and uncertainty made it impossible or near impossible to meet.

This imaginative visualization of the night and its cultural spaces recalls geographer Doreen Massey's concept of 'space–time', in which space is embedded in temporality. As Massey noted, 'both space and landscape could be imagined as provisionally intertwined simultaneities of ongoing, unfinished stories. Space, as a dimension, cuts through such trajectories, but not to stabilise them into a surface; rather space is imbued with time' (Massey 2006: 21). Echoing Williams' (2008) considerations about the practices of territorialization with which the night has often been associated, Massey's conceptualization seems to poignantly convey how, during the pandemic, the arts captured this complex entanglement of histories of oppression and marginalization, as well as the resistance and self-expression with which the night has been associated. It resonates in *Bacurau*'s prescient evocation of the plight of millions under COVID-19, particularly those at the mercy of inadequate healthcare provision and even state-sponsored necropolitics, which was to happen in Brazil.

As *Bacurau*'s night scenes move into the daytime, the film suggests a continuity between the drama and nightmarish atmosphere that the cover of darkness provides by punctuating the storytelling with instances of haunting. Fleeting human figures are glimpsed in the background, empty rocking chairs are eerily in motion on a house veranda and the apparition of the deceased black town matriarch Carmelita (played by the iconic African Brazilian singer Lia de Itamaracá) appears; these all contribute to the building of an atmosphere of haunting, in which the current authorities' playing with life and death echoes the crimes of the country's historical past, of undemocratic leadership, extractivist violence, slavery and its legacy, denial of civil rights, among them.

Conclusion

To conclude, I would argue that there is something of the *terreiro* in Bacurau's revolt against the official politics of death. The extreme violence into which the plot descends remains problematic, but this is something to which the film itself draws attention. As mercenary leader Michael meets his unsavoury end, he yells to his captors that 'this is only the beginning', a warning that wonton bloodshed does not bring resolution. Yet, the film is striking in how it envisages the possibility of resistance in the face of historic injustice. As the world faced the devastation of the COVID-19 pandemic, the situation also provided audiences in more affluent parts of the world with a reminder that, for some, the recent catastrophe is but a new instalment in a long history of health and social injustice. Yet it also imagines a space–time under cover of darkness where future possibilities can be envisioned in this re-encounter with 'the plague'.

NOTE
1. All translations from Portuguese are by the chapter's author, unless otherwise stated.

REFERENCES
Backstein, K. (2020), 'Bacurau', *Cineaste*, 45:3, pp. 52–53.

Bentes, I. (2019), 'Bacurau e a síntese do Brasil brutal', *Revista Cult*, 29 August.

Brandão, A. and Sousa, R. Lira de (2020), 'Bodylands: Para além da invisibilidade lésbica no cinema: Brincando com água', *Rebeca – Revista Brasileira de Estudos de Cinema e Audiovisual*, 9:2, pp. 98–118.

Chazkel, A. (2017), 'The invention of night: Visibility and violence after dark in Rio de Janeiro', in G. Santamaría and D. Carey (eds), *The Publics and Politics of Violence in Latin America*, Norman, Ok: University of Oklahoma Press, pp. 143–58.

Conde, M. (2020), 'Brazil in the time of coronavirus', *Geopolítica(s): Revista de estudios sobre espacio y poder*, 11, pp. 239–49.

Dunn, N. and Edensor, T. (2020), *Rethinking Darkness: Cultures, Histories, Practices*, London: Routledge.

Ferreira, C. O. and Nafafé, J. L. (2021), 'Resistência, necropolítica e fantasias de vingança: Bacurau (2019), de Kleber Mendonça Filho e Juliano Dornelles', *Rebeca – Revista Brasileira de Estudos de Cinema e Audiovisual*, 10:2, pp. 244–76.

Film at Lincoln Centre (2020), 'The directors of Bacurau & Sônia Braga on the making of their Brazilian thriller', YouTube, 6 March, https://www.youtube.com/watch?v=-z51vOSxus8. Accessed 19 December 2022.

Fischer, M. M. J. (2021), 'Bacurau flies at dusk: Film, viral cultural politics, Covid-19, hauntings, and futures', *Anuário Antropológico*, 46:1, pp. 166–89.

Gomes, P. H. (2020), '"Não sou coveiro, tá?", diz Bolsonaro ao responder sobre mortos por coronavirus', *O Globo*, 20 April, https://g1.globo.com/politica/noticia/2020/04/20/nao-sou-coveiro-ta-diz-bolsonaro-ao-responder-sobre-mortos-por-coronavirus.ghtml. Accessed 25 March 2024.

Ikeda, M. (2020), 'The ambuities of Badura', *Film Quarterly*, 74:2, pp. 81–83.

Lefebvre, H. ([1974] 1991), *The Production of Space* (trans. D. Nicholson-Smith), Oxford: Blackwell.

Massey, D. (2006), 'Landscape as a provocation: Reflections on moving mountains', *Journal of Material Culture*, 11:1&2, 33–48.

Mattos, R. (2019), 'Tropicalismo e canção engajada no filme Bacurau', *Esquerda Online*, 29 September, Tropicalismo e canção engajada no filme BacurauEsquerda Onlinehttps://esquerdaonline.com.br › tr. Accessed 25 March 2024.

Mbembe, A. (2019), *Necropolitics* (trans. Steven Corcoran), Durham, NC: Duke University Press.

Mendonça Filho, K. (2019), 'Kleber Mendonça Filho: "Não fiz um panfleto". Interview with Molica F. and Motta, B', *Revista Veja*, 29 September, https://veja.abril.com.br/cultura/kleber-mendonca-filho-bacurau/https://veja.abril.com.br/cultura/kleber-mendonca-filho-bacurau/. Accessed 25 March 2024.

Mittelman, D. M. (2022), 'White horror in Bacurau', *Romance Quarterly*, 20, pp. 1–20.

Palmer, R. (2000), *Cultures of Darkness: Night Travels in the Histories of Transgression (from Medieval to Modern)*, New York: Monthly Review Press.

Rubinstein, B. (2020), 'Drag artist Silvero Pereira on getting blood-soaked in *Bacurau*', *Interview Magazine*, 6 March, https://www.interviewmagazine.com/film/silvero-pereira-bacurau. Accessed 20 December 2022.

Williams, R. (2008), 'Night spaces: Darkness, deterritorialization, and social control', *Space and Culture*, 11:4, pp. 514–32.

12

A Pandemic Crisis Seen from the Screen: A Reflection on Pandemic Imagination

Anna Nacher, Søren Bro Pold and Scott Rettberg

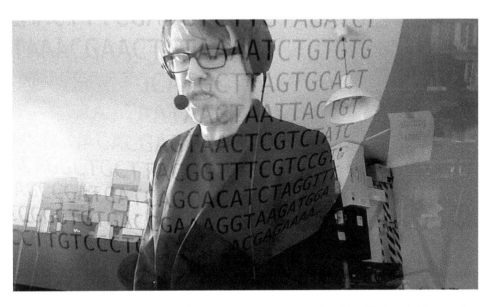

FIGURE 12.1: Jörg Piringer: *Covid-19 genome* poem, screenshot from Piringer's 'Quarantine TV'. Courtesy of the artist.

Since the COVID-19 pandemic faded in early 2022, the agenda has been overtaken by other major issues, such as the wars in Ukraine and Gaza, and this has led to a certain tiredness if not bare repression of the pandemic experience. However, we believe it is important to revisit the cultural experience of the pandemic not only to reflect on how it challenged us and our societies but also to point out alternatives that are still relevant now, even if other problems have occurred (see Figure 12.1). In fact, the very experience of the pandemic as a hyperobject might be worth reflecting on, as we will attempt to do below, in order to understand and deal with other continuing hyperobject crises such as racism, inequality and climate destruction (Morton 2013). Our focus in the following will be on our research on electronic literature, digital artists and the pandemic, which we will present below, including a focus on our chosen work by the artist Ben Grosser *The Endless Doomscroller*, which will be put in relation to other works from our exhibition, collection and documentary.

During the COVID-19 pandemic, we became acquainted with medical scientists, epidemiologists and statisticians, but even after the pandemic we still miss a clearer understanding of the cultural, existential and epistemological questions of the pandemic and more than a year of isolated screen reality. Cultural life and institutions seem to be the least prioritised after opening society, even if crises hit hard within these fields. Nevertheless, cultural and collective processing of the pandemic is taking place, and this is important for both contemporary and future preparedness for coping with pandemics and larger crises. The German scholar of memory studies, Astrid Errl, points to how we were unprepared in Europe in 2020 when COVID-19 arrived because we were largely spared from recent epidemics such as Ebola, Zika virus, MERS and SARS, and because AIDS HIV mainly hit a minority group. Even though 50,000,000 people died during the Spanish Flu (1918–19) pandemic, it has largely been forgotten, perhaps because of its entanglement with the aftermath of the First World War and other epidemics like tuberculosis, as well as its lack of narrativity, tellability and canonical visual art. Compared to the medieval plague, 'the Spanish Flu was "not sufficiently imagined". As it was not a "pandemic imagined", it did not turn into a "pandemic remembered"' (Erll 2020a: 865, 2020b). This leads us to ask how our current pandemic will be imagined and remembered.

Digital art and electronic literature have, since their beginnings, explored new and alternative modes of narrativity and visuality, including discussions about the very foundation of narration and visuality in digital media marked by interaction, coded and algorithmic infrastructures, networks, etc., resulting in genres such as combinatory poetics, hypertext fiction, interactive fiction and poetry and network writing (Rettberg 2019). Exploring the aesthetics of digital art related to the pandemic is relevant in order to discuss how to understand, process and cope with it. This might also be relevant for similar crises in the digital age. By virtue of its artistic medium of expression, digital art reflects on life on and behind the screen, including how we are increasingly governed by interfaces, corporate platforms and software. The pandemic crisis has been a climax in the age of corporate meta-interfaces and platform culture (Andersen and Pold 2018; Gillespie 2010) in which many have carried out their work, social life, education and cultural activities entirely behind and through screens. If the current pandemic had happened 30 years ago, all these experiences would have been different and much more difficult. People have learned to take advantage of all the tools and services of platform culture – as the skyrocketing stock values of corporate platform companies like Amazon, Facebook, Google and Zoom during the pandemic demonstrate – however, there has also been increased awareness of the shortcomings, problems and damage caused by these platforms. Discussions of everything from Zoom fatigue, how platforms are squeezing and even strangling their content producers, how social media are damaging to public discourse and democracy, to issues of surveillance capitalism and the carbon emission of cloud computing have entered the public sphere, and there is a greater understanding emerging of the costs of our 'free' participation in activities on platforms.

Consequently, we set out to explore the aesthetics, narrativity and use of media in electronic literature and digital art related to COVID-19. Beginning in the spring of 2020, shortly after the first lockdown, we began exploring how digital art and electronic literature (e-lit) relate to the pandemic through online discussions, a questionnaire and a conference roundtable, which took place on 17 July 2020 at the Electronic Literature Organization's (ELO) 2020 conference and is well documented.[1] This initial work led to the 'Electronic Literature and COVID-19' project (funded by DARIAH-EU) and a call for projects for the exhibition *Covid E-lit – Digital Art from the Pandemic*, which opened on 1 May 2021 with 24 works chosen through peer review which was presented at an opening and the ELO 2021 conference.[2]

Our respondents were primarily from North America and Europe. We also created the research collection on the ELMCIP knowledge base that collects works reflecting on the pandemic.[3] Furthermore, during March and April, we conducted recorded interviews through video conference (Zoom) with eighteen artists who were responsible for thirteen different works. Each interview lasted about 45–60 minutes as part of the project. The interviewed artists were chosen first because their work was interesting and of high artistic quality, and second, with consideration of approaching a diversity of themes, approaches, gender, ethnicity and geography. The interviewed artists and works were: Alex Saum: *Room #3* (San Francisco), Jody Zellen: *Ghost City, Avenue S* (Boston, NY, Los Angeles), Ben Grosser: *Endless Doomscroller* (Urbana Champaign), Annie Abrahams: *Pandemic Encounter* (NL, Montpellier, FR), Sharon Daniel and Erik Loyer: *Exposed* (Santa Barbara, LA), Mark Sample: *Content Moderator Sim* (Davidson, North Carolina), Mark Marino and Family: *Coronation* (Los Angeles), Giulia Carla-Rossi: *The British Library Simulator* (London), Bilal Mohammed: *Lost Inside: A Digital Inquiry* (San Diego),

Xtine Burrough: *I got up* (Dallas), Giselle Beiguelman: *Coronario* (São Paulo), Jörg Piringer: *QuarantineTV + Virus genome* (Vienna), and Judd Morrisey, Abraham Avnisan and Mark Jeffery: *The Tenders: Embrasures in the Fort's Collapse* (Chicago). From the open call, we did get a majority of works from the United States, which is still noticeable in the list of interviewees above, though we chose to include some from outside of the United States to mitigate this imbalance. The overweight of the US-based works might be partly coincidental but might also have something to do with the fact that the call was released as part of the ELO 2021 conference, even though ELO has lately aimed and succeeded to include artists and researchers from outside of the United States, including from Europe, South East Asia, Africa, etc. ELO was founded in the United States and is probably still best incorporated into North American academic traditions and literary departments, whereas the field of digital arts in Europe and Asia is oriented more towards media art festivals, such as Ars Electronica (Linz) or Transmediale (Berlin) and museums, such as Zentrum für Kunst und Medien, Karlsruhe (ZKM). Even though these fields overlap significantly, there still seems to be a wall separating them; hence, our conscious use of both electronic literature and digital art in our titles and texts.

The interviews were conducted as semi-structured (Leavy and Brinkmann 2014) with questions related to (1) a description of and motivation behind the work, (2) the choice of genres and literary, aesthetic and narrative strategies, (3) reflections on the pandemic from its outbreak to the time of the interviews one year later, (4) reflections on making e-lit and digital art during the age of platform culture and online life, (5) relations to the artistic and social community during the pandemic, (6) the relation of the pandemic to other current crises, (7) the physical environment and the effects being homebound during the lockdown and (8) their localized experience of the pandemic.[4] The interviews formed the basis of the 44-minute documentary *Covid E-Lit: Digital Art During the Pandemic*, which premiered at the 2021 Oslo International Poetry Festival and is publicly available on the open web (Nacher et al. 2022). Libraries (including the Roskilde Library, Bergen Library and The British Library) are also screening the film and including it in their collections.[5]

Obviously, many activities and artworks are dealing with the pandemic around the world, and we do not claim to be able to obtain a full overview of all this.[6] However, through our method with conference roundtables and panels, an open call, interviews, questionnaires and open presentations of material and findings, we believe that we can claim a structured, qualitative procedure and collection of material within the global community of electronic literature and neighbouring fields. Hopefully, this secures some basis and validity for our observations, though it is the case that the pandemic has been experienced individually as well as collectively and in many different contexts and societies across the world. Even within small, rich countries, such as Denmark or Norway, there are large differences between the experiences of a fairly well-off middle class comfortably sequestered in their own houses and gardens and students living in dormitories or migrants living closely together in community apartments. Furthermore, the differences between individual experiences in countries where the spread of infection has been fairly under control and others, where it has not been sufficiently contained which led to political turmoil (such as the United States, Brazil, India, etc.) are important, as are the differences between people working at front-line jobs (such as nurses or bus drivers) and office workers working from home (cf. also Erll 2020a: 863; Markham et al. 2020: 2). Even if our pool of interviewees included people from different countries and ethnicities, by focusing on artists who were also often academics, our demography overrepresented people working from home in relative safety. This aspect is addressed in the interview by Mark Sample, where he, in a remarkably self-critical way, looks back at his work from the beginning of the pandemic, *The Infinite Catalog of Crushed Dreams*:

> When I look back at *The Infinite Catalog of Crushed Dreams*, I almost cringe at how middle-class Anglo-centric, American-centric it is. And partly that's because I based it on my own experiences and what was being filtered through me, to me, through friends and family. But, on the other hand, it just seems very ignorant of what we now know to be the really disparate impact of the virus itself and the economic shutdown, shutdowns on different groups of people. So that the kind of people who are mostly in *Infinite Catalog* are people who are probably still doing OK, versus, you know, like Latinx or African Americans or people in other countries, that now there's this kind of vaccine disparity that we see unfolding, I feel like my piece doesn't capture all those realities of the pandemic that we now know.
>
> (Sample 2021: n.pag.)

However, in our exhibition and as part of our interviews, we do have several works and artists that represent vulnerable populations, such as Sharon Daniel and Erik Loyer's *Exposed* (about inmates exposed to COVID in the US incarceration system), Giselle Beiguelman's *Coronario* (about how the pandemic-related language was controlled in Brazil by the Bolsonaro's government and Google) or Bilal Mohammed's *Lost Inside: A Digital Inquiry* (which includes reflections on experiencing the pandemic from a minority perspective).

Unrepresentability and monumentality

As pointed out by Astrid Erll, the experience of the Spanish Flu in 1918/19 has 'remained unremembered', even though it killed more people than the First World

War and Second World War put together (Erll 2020a, 2020b: 47). Just as there are virtually no monuments to the Spanish Flu, it is difficult to imagine monuments to COVID-19 beyond the many graphs and statistics we have been relentlessly exposed to. Erll indeed points out that

> Covid-19 is the first global pandemic of the digital age. In terms of archives (including worldwide digital information about case numbers and the circulation of personal experiences via social media), there will be an abundance of sources for future collective memory.
>
> (Erll 2020a, 2020b: 49)

In this sense, the pandemic has left its mark online, whereas in the physical world, it has mainly been marked by a lack of traffic, people on the street, pollution and urban life and culture in general. The American artist Ben Grosser has made a continuous visualization on Instagram, almost as an illustration of how one can (not) imagine a suitable monument during the pandemic (see Figure 12.2). Based on the scale of the 9/11 monument in New York, he outlined how much space a monument of COVID-19 would require. The nearly 3000 killed in 2001 are

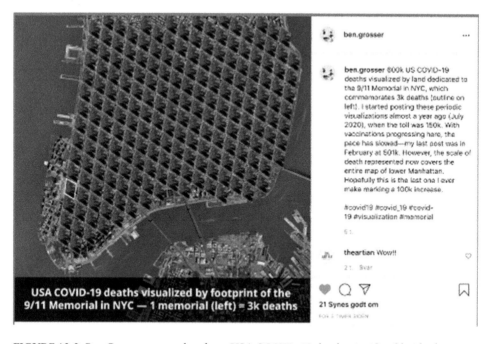

FIGURE 12.2: Ben Grosser: screenshot from *USA COVID-19 deaths visualized by the footprint of the 9/11 Memorial in NYC* (Instagram). Courtesy of the artist.

commemorated in the footprint the World Trade Center towers occupied, and if this scale were to be followed, then at the moment of writing, the more than 600,000 dead in the United States alone would take up 200 blocks in Manhattan's grid, corresponding to all of Lower Manhattan.

It seems that, to get to a cultural understanding of the pandemic, it is necessary to recognize the ways it disrupts our established frameworks of understanding the world. It is difficult to recognize the significance of major crises while they are happening, especially those that mark a major shift. There are many indications that this is the case here and that the pandemic will be seen at the level of other pivotal moments, such as the fall of the Berlin Wall, the emergence of digital culture and 9/11. Similar to how the Belarus Nobel Prize Laureate Svetlana Alexievich describes the situation for the people on the ground in Ukraine and Belarus in *Chernobyl Prayer*, it is a new kind of crisis that is somewhat invisible and is difficult to comprehend and predict the effects of; this disrupts traditional understandings of coherent time and space. The crisis cannot be localized or enclosed, and we cannot know when it is finally over or to what degree it is a sign of a new condition for living on the planet:

> In so many ways, the issue is massive and, at the same time, microscopic. These scales compete with each other as explanations for the ethnographic question: 'what is going on here?' They compete for our attention. They are simultaneously dialogic, oppositional, chaotic/inchoate, both/and.
>
> (Markham et al. 2020: 2)

It is perhaps no coincidence that commemoration of the victims seems to be an ambivalent undertaking and while the private and city-level attempts proliferate, the broader, national or international initiatives are stalling – as if the Covid pandemic (once it's over) were to be removed from public memory (Mooallem 2023).[7] In this sense, the pandemic is best understood as belonging to the class of what Timothy Morton calls hyperobjects: phenomena such as global warming, nuclear radiation, etc. that are 'massively distributed entities that can be thought and computed but not directly touched or seen. The simultaneous unavailability yet reality of the hyperobject requires a radical new form of thinking to cope with it' (Morton 2013: 39).

Michael Taussig compares the pandemic urban space to Giorgio de Chirico's melancholy paintings of Roman arcades and empty streets, which he describes as 'capturing the aura Walter Benjamin found in Eugène Atget's photographs of Paris streets likewise without people' (Taussig 2021: 33). Interestingly, Atget's photographs were remade by Mauricio Lima during the lockdown in spring 2020, striking an atmosphere that many can recognize from walking in empty urban streets through the lockdown, where most of the normal life, functions and institutions of the city were paused, diverted and left as empty shells (Nossiter 2020). Taussig sees potential for redemption in this through its re-enchanting of a disenchanted nature that has led to the climate and biodiversity crisis and he thinks that we need a new kind of aesthetics and experience:

> But what the question opens up is the thought that, with global meltdown, we now live in a reenchanted universe for which the aesthetic of a dark surrealism is relevant. It is a mutating reality of metamorphic sublimity that never lets you know what is real and what is not. Born from WWI, there is a lot of Dada here too, with its shock effects and montage. We were told the bourgeoisie had gotten bored with that. But now, has not Dada and surrealism returned with a vengeance? Before, it was avant-garde subsiding into history. But now, with the reenchantment of nature, history is subsiding into Dada.
> (Taussig 2021: 35–36)

Taussig mentions the shock effects and montage of Dada, which we will get back to below. He follows Benjamin in arguing for the relevance of a new perception, a re-enchantment or what Benjamin calls a 'literarization of the conditions of life', which points to changes in our epistemic understanding of our surroundings, environment and our place in this (Benjamin 1999: 527).

Related to the portrayal of the conditions of life and the deserted urban public, American net artist Jody Zellen has made *Avenue S* a new part of her enduring net art piece *Ghost City* (see Figure 12.3). She calls it a 'pandemic journal' and a 'response to what's around', which is simultaneously 'comical, tragic and humorous' in its ways of showing empty streets with lonely stick figures endlessly spinning on treadmills or trying to move on in difficult settings. It portrays people mechanically controlled by their environment as an allegory of life during the pandemic, but perhaps parallel to Taussig's hope for a re-enchantment, there are also beautiful moments that show people's reactions through, for example, drawings on the street or moments of protest and demonstrations such as Black Lives Matter. The piece expresses a general, specific impersonal, non-auratic beauty through its visual expression and societal perspective. It shows us faceless people behind masks who are threatened by anxiety and angst in persistent patterns, but the patterns have a sense of beauty. It includes many animations of people spinning in repeated circles, which are both tragic and meditative:

> there's a lot of kind of spinning in circles, you know, because I think that's technically how we feel, how I feel. And again, it was sort of the hope that how I feel can resonate with how other people are feeling now.
> (Zellen 2021: n.pag.)

A PANDEMIC CRISIS SEEN FROM THE SCREEN

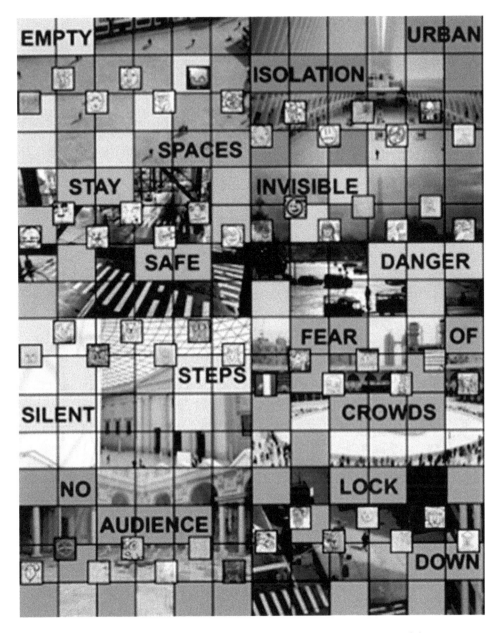

FIGURE 12.3: Jody Zellen: screenshot from *Ghost City, Avenue S*. Courtesy of the artist.

The piece is, as Zellen states, 'kind of narrative', though 'certainly not linear' but rather circular 'so the very last page always goes back to the very first page [...] it always takes you around and around like you're getting lost in the city from which you can't escape'. *Avenue S* marks a return to net art for Zellen as 'a kind of public art' during a pandemic where the public became digital through commercial platforms and where the urban public is deserted. Its collages become like cave paintings from the present to the future, or in Siegfried Kracauer's sense, pandemic mass ornaments, showing us a 'literarization of the conditions of life' during the pandemic.[8] In this sense, *Avenue S* is an allegory of the pandemic, showing what is not immediately represented: how the biopolitics of the pandemic with all its statistical measures create a different society where humans are not placed at centre stage but are figures in an urban and environmental scenography.

Pandemic language, discourse and narrative economy

The discourse during the pandemic has been influenced by the many new words that have come along with it, and some of these words have been part of both an ideological and algorithmic battle zone. The Brazilian artist Giselle Beiguelman created a hypertext essay called 'Coronário / Coronary' based on 25 corona-related words, which reflects on how language is affected by the pandemic (see Figure 12.4). However, the work also shows how language use is monitored by platforms, demonstrated in the work through a heat map where the words are coloured by click rate as a parallel to how Google or Facebook registers user behaviour. *Coronary* has a special focus on Brazil, which has been hit very hard by the pandemic and by Jair Bolsonaro's incompetence in dealing with it. It contains words such as

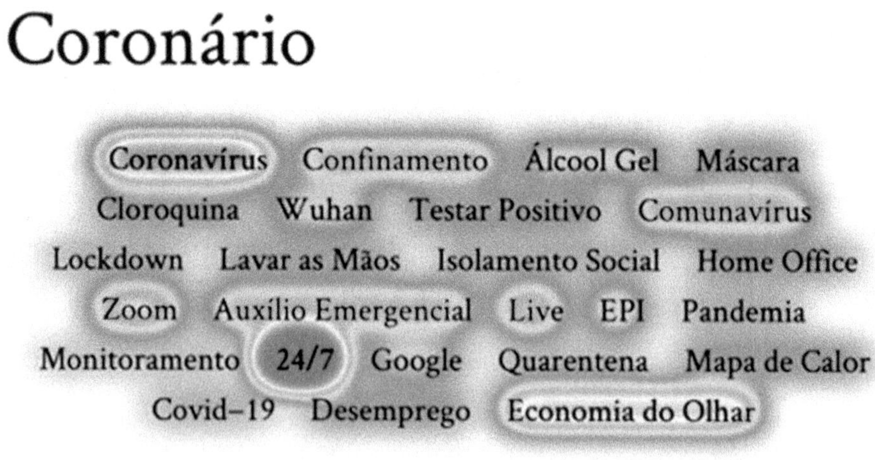

Coronário

Coronavírus   Confinamento   Álcool Gel   Máscara
Cloroquina   Wuhan   Testar Positivo   Comunavírus
Lockdown   Lavar as Mãos   Isolamento Social   Home Office
Zoom   Auxílio Emergencial   Live   EPI   Pandemia
Monitoramento   24/7   Google   Quarentena   Mapa de Calor
Covid–19   Desemprego   Economia do Olhar

FIGURE 12.4: Screenshot from *Coronário* by Giselle Beiguelman. Courtesy of the artist.

'Communavirus' created by Bolsonaro's foreign minister to link coronavirus with communism in the style of Donald Trump's 'China virus', and a word like 'mask' changes its contextual meaning from being associated with carnival to quarantine.

When we asked her about her choice of aesthetic strategy and genre, Giselle Beiguelman stated how the work is related to the political situation in Brazil and the development of new words and discourse:

> One year ago, at the beginning of the coronavirus pandemic […], our ambassador, the minister of foreign affairs, stated that there was no coronavirus. What we have in the world is a pandemic of communa-virus that the virus came from China and it was inoculating spies. […] This was just the beginning. And this discourse I was looking about, what does it mean, […] and I was doing a search on Google Trends to measure the impact of these words […]. And it was a little bit disappointing, because, yes, it was something exclusive of us in Portuguese. […] And then the Google Trends suggests at the same time, well, if you are searching for these, maybe you can compare with these. Suddenly, there was a constellation of words that we never used before, like alcohol gel and pandemic. And so, I decided to do more objective research and work with it, in the logic of the Google Trends, the Google Trends always organizes the results in groups of 25 words. […] So it was clear that language was the skin, the first level of a very deep change, social, political and cultural that we were, by then discovering; now it's becoming our new normal. And then I decided to make this reading clear through an interface that registered the attention that each word receives from the public.
>
> (Beiguelman 2021: n.pag.)

As it becomes clear, *Coronary* is a work about language, how language is ideologically controlled by the Bolsonaro regime and how this is reinforced by surveillance technologies in a situation that has been integrated with a conflictual political situation in Brazil that has been carried out concerning the pandemic and the Bolsonaro government's (lack of) reaction to it. In our interview, Beiguelman further explains how this is related to Brazilian social conflicts and people living in favelas without the necessary space for social isolation or the resources to stay isolated, which has led to an increase in the number of people living on the street. During a period in which information visualization became the primary mode of communicating the immensity of the crisis, Beiguelman used the vernacular of visualization to communicate the weaponization of language as a discourse of power.

The control of discourse through platforms such as Google and Facebook has in general led to pressure on public discourse. Even if sensationalist news is not new, it is now algorithmically proliferated by social media, resulting in a favouring of extreme voices with a lack of nuances and in some cases even conspiracies, which are growing out of the pent-up emotions after more than a year in social isolation. *The Endless Doomscroller* by Ben Grosser shows how the algorithmic feed mechanisms of social media, combined with click-bait headlines and a populace stuck online, form a 'perfect yet evil marriage' promoting a desire for more engagement without bringing satisfaction (see Figure 12.5) (Grosser 2021a). *The Endless Doomscroller* demonstrates how this combination of clickbait and social media creates a plot machine without closure that creates engagement rather than knowledge, which is perfectly in line with the social media business model. Users get an endless scroll of bad news, which is never too concrete or precise, but enables endless scrolling of ominous headlines.

An affective compulsion to consume ambient information supersedes a connection to a specific incident or even to reality. As pointed out by Grosser, *The Endless Doomscroller*'s primary technique is one of reduction by how it 'distils news and social media sites down to their barest most generalized messages and interface conventions', such as simplified negative headlines and the infinite scroll interface

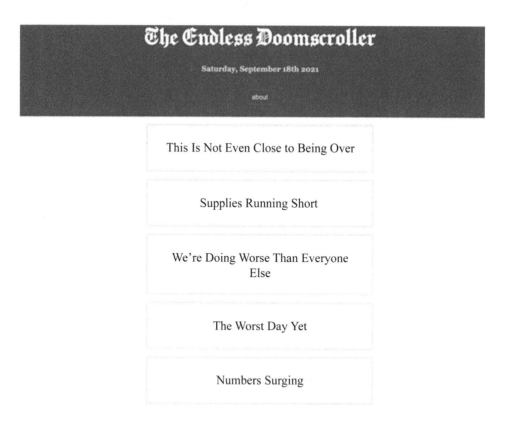

FIGURE 12.5: Screenshot from *The Endless Doomscroller* by Ben Grosser. Courtesy of the artist.

of social media. He characterizes the infinite scroll interface common to social media as a 'minimalist hiding [...] of the datafication, monitoring and profiling going on in cloud computing infrastructures behind its immediate, minimalist user-interface' which keeps the user in a WHILE loop where the practical stop condition becomes 'something akin to a fatal exception in computing', such as when the user falls asleep or the device runs out of power (Grosser 2021a: 3). Grosser concludes, 'Through these tactics, *The Endless Doomscroller* deconstructs the doomscrolling metainterface, revealing how it is changing what and how we read in the digital and pandemic age' (Grosser 2021a: 6). It is a work that demonstrates and consequently makes people aware of the mechanisms behind the metainterface. In our interview, Grosser mentions how he was inspired by his being 'stuck in a pattern of just continually scrolling and scanning' and taking his own experience as a starting point he hopes to

> help people develop their own critical lens on what it means to be a user of a platform. That is a relationship that is, from the platform's perspective, a hyper-designed, hyper-analyzed relationship that is all about the production of certain kinds of behavior from the user.
>
> (Ben Grosser 2021b: n.pag.)

Consequently, *The Endless Doomscroller* explores the pandemic plot machine, its algorithms, interface and infrastructure from the user interface perspective – it critically reflects on how users are subject to the pandemic plot machine, which with the above suggestion by Taussig and by Tristan Tzara's 'To make a dadaist poem' in mind can characterize as digital dadaism.

The American artist Mark Sample has made a parallel work with *Content Moderator Sim* that moves the perspective behind the immediate user interface. It is a game that simulates the working environment for social media content moderators who, on a tight piecework schedule, sort all the materials that have been marked as offensive by users or algorithms. In the game, users are presented with repeated examples, with the option of either allowing or blocking, stressed by the tight pressure of time. Often it is impossible within the given time to determine whether it is expressions of marginalized groups, coarse jokes or actual racism and violent hate speech. The game clearly reflects the stressful role of being the editor who must muck out the trash of social media, and, according to the interview we did with Mark Sample, it is realistic in the sense that he 'interwove into the game various rationales from Facebook's own handbooks that it gives its content moderators about when something is acceptable or not'. Ultimately, the game portrays how the human content moderators are themselves almost turned into algorithms by this interface to gauge these expressions: 'the content moderator humans are just placeholders until AI is sophisticated enough to do this work'. The process is an example of human computation in which human labour – in this case, ethical judgment – is simplified to being just one step in a computational process, directed by an algorithm rather than by human intelligence. Later, Sample continues:

> I was trying to capture almost a clinically detached point of view, like the player character's voice is pretty detached describing these things until there's like one or two moments when it breaks through, like the actual emotion punched through. I was trying to capture that sense of it's almost like it's the paid version of doom scrolling.
>
> (Sample 2021: n.pag.)

In this way, Grosser and Sample show two sides of how the interface that was our primary social platform during the lockdown is constructed and how its narrative plot machinery is staged, including exploring the architecture of the interface scenography as well as the people working backstage. Both works also contain narratives partly generated by algorithms and portray how we are caught in the discourse platforms of social media. As mentioned above, at the beginning of the pandemic, Mark Sample made another work, *The Infinite Catalog of Crushed Dreams*, where an endless list of cancellations is generated under the heading 'The pandemic hit and then'. It is easy to recognize the experience of how everything was cancelled without mercy by a pandemic that was more intrusive than we, in our wildest imaginations, would have thought a few months before. The generative algorithm simulates the effect of a virus over which we have no control, and it works worryingly well as a relentless narrator of the drama of the pandemic.

The most relentless and least human digital narrator is presented by Austrian artist and sound poet Jörg Piringer's *Covid-19 genome* sound poem, in which a computer voice reads out the entire original virus genetic sequence at a fast pace. The poem is 13 minutes and 27 seconds of variants of TTTCGATC, and it draws attention to the fact that the virus itself can be represented as a form of language – for example, the word CAT is included several times and, as Piringer jokingly points out, cats provide a good basis for viral spread in a platform culture – but a language we still struggle to understand, including in its variations and mutations. As Piringer points out in our interview:

> The algorithms that scientists used to analyse genomes in general, are text algorithms, in fact. So, there's a kind of small section of computer science that is called […] stringology, which is about strings, character strings. And what they do is find patterns in strings and analyse them. And that's actually what we as artists do. And especially when you work with data and transform it into literature, that's what

you do when you work with computers, and they do it as well. So, it is kind of very closely related. They don't see it as literature, but you could see it as literature I think.
(Piringer 2021: n.pag.)

All of these works point to how language in the context of software platforms has been shaped in an algorithmic power struggle that has also shaped us. This power struggle includes technological, commercial, political, national and international actors, and it ranges from the very words the pandemic is presented with, as exemplified by Beiguelman, to the way they are presented and plotted in technological, political and commercial platforms, as demonstrated by Grosser and Sample, and to the way that the virus itself is represented and treated as coded letters and strings, including in DNA sequencing to develop vaccines or finding mutations, as explored by Piringer. In general, it points to a semioticization process which, combined with increased computation, leads to a pandemic discourse economy where language becomes power (as in who controls the rhetoric), capital (as in who controls our attention) and even biology through genetic virus code that we struggle to understand but might reflect on as/through literature. As N. Katherine Hayles points out, the novel coronavirus is posthuman in that it is 'oblivious to human intentions, desires, and motives', but also in the more technical way that humans and viruses have adopted diametrically opposed evolutionary strategies of complexity versus simplicity, though viruses are still an important part of biological evolution and reproduction. As Hayles puts it, 'It screams at jet engine volume that we are interdependent not only with each other but also with the entire ecology of the earth' (Hayles 2021: 68, 70).

What are the poetics of this pandemic discourse economy? Clearly, it shares the allegorical dark surrealism pointed out above, of how our language and representations are enmeshed in capitalist processes that cannot be immediately seen by the individual, but which need interfaces like the ones produced by Beiguelman, Grosser, Sample and Piringer that have detached, algorithmic narrators.[9] However, these works also point towards the use of lists, like Grosser and Sample's litany of litanies. Mark Sample comments on this in our interview:

Yeah, *The Infinite Catalog of Crushed Dreams*. And it's this kind of infinite scrolling piece. The more you scroll, you just see these lists and lists of different people and scenarios that have just been utterly broken by the coronavirus shutdown. And I was trying to capture that sense that I was feeling at the time, which is like a year ago now. So last March, I think it's when I started working on it, that feeling of, I was seeing it in my own kids and seeing it in my students, like prom was being cancelled. That concert they trained, and rehearsed for months for the play was canceled, all those trips that were canceled. So, I am just trying to capture that sense of loss. And you just keep scrolling and scrolling and there's, I haven't figured out the mathematics behind it, but the chances of things repeating themselves, it's like it's in the billions, one in billions of things repeating.

(Sample 2021: n.pag.)

As Sample points out, the endless litanies represent a loss of control related to the virus' obliviousness to human intentions that Hayles describes; however, as pointed out by Grosser, it also becomes a mode of control enacted by the 'perfect yet evil marriage' by click-bait news and social media in a new kind of brutal digital dadaism, and Beiguelman even points to something similar as a way of controlling language by Google and the Bolsonaro regime. Hence, we see a semantic drift or even a drift of signifiers, that becomes apparent in a situation where people are struggling to make sense of the pandemic. Perhaps this drift is the current that we navigate in, trying to keep our heads above water in our individual and collective sense-making process (Nacher 2021).

Post-pandemic poetics

To conclude on the poetics of the pandemic, we have observed issues related to the representation and realism of the pandemic. As written above, with Morton, Taussig, Benjamin and Kracauer we have characterized this realism as an allegorical dark surrealism aimed at dealing with the unrepresentability of the pandemic hyperobject. Part of the unrepresentability relates to the fact that the human is decentered, if not killed, by an invisible virus, made visible through statistical control measures and biopolitics such as shown in the works of Ben Grosser (in his *USA COVID-19 deaths*[...]) and Jody Zellen. Furthermore, this kind of realism is achieved and narrated through detached, dadaist and brutal algorithmic narrators as reflected in the works by Giselle Beiguelman, Ben Grosser, Mark Sample and Jörg Piringer, enforced by economic, discursive, technologically plotted and biopolitically coded powers. As we argued with Astrid Erll (2020a, 2020b), COVID-19 is the first pandemic of the digital age and we experienced it to a large degree through digital platforms.

It is perhaps not strange that we are happy with the pandemic being over and that there are plenty of new crises to be occupied with. However, the combination of digital modelling, platformization and real-world effects does not make the pandemic unreal or virtual, but a genuine experience of a crisis related to hyperobjects – after all we rarely observed the disease directly but mainly through statistics and predictions that confined our living space and social lives such as the endless generated list of cancellations in Mark Sample's *The Infinite Catalog*.

Consequently, the COVID-19 pandemic brought a moment of reflection on the many seemingly unsolvable contemporary crises, including the climate crisis, gender and social inequality, racism, colonialism, as well as social and economic harms inflicted by platform capitalism. The experience of the hyperobject of the pandemic crisis allowed us to relate to other major crises that are also part of the works mentioned above and in our documentary, thus also opening up the space for empathy and hope for change. This reflective moment was dimmed in 2022, with the war in Ukraine urgently requiring a swift response. However, the new crises did not extinguish the old ones. Therefore, there is a need to revisit the reflections inspired by the pandemic lockdown to prompt the potential of change, even if filled with loss. In this way, electronic literature and digital art can potentially help us to better cope with hyperobjects beyond our immediate control and provide us with a means to construct a collective imaginary of our platformed present and its crises, hence learning the strategies for, as insightfully framed by Christos Lynteris following Julietta Singh, 'unthinking mastery' of human beings (Lynteris 2019: 120; Singh 2017). It is noteworthy that both accounts of how humans would need to bid farewell to the supposed control of other agencies present in the world have been offered before the COVID-19 pandemic and were based on research into the cultural patterns established after the previous pandemic episodes in human history, which only further emphasizes the need for more robust reflection around the recent wave of viral intervention in the course of human history.

ACKNOWLEDGEMENTS
Thanks to all the artists who participated and made this work possible. The project is co-funded by DARIAH-EU Digital Research Infrastructure for the Arts and Humanities.

NOTES
1. The roundtable is documented here: https://stars.library.ucf.edu/elo2020/live/roundtables/7/. Accessed 14 March 2024.
2. The exhibition *Covid E-lit – Digital Art from the Pandemic* is available at https://www.eliterature.org/elo2021/covid/. Accessed 14 March 2024. Our panel 'Post(?) Pandemic Prose: Preliminary Findings of the Covid E-Lit' project was presented 27 May 2021 at the Platform Post(?) Pandemic ELO 2021 conference and a recording of it is available here: https://vimeo.com/555698083. Accessed 14 March 2024.
3. Pandemic E-Lit at *Elmcip Knowledge Base* is available here: https://elmcip.net/research-collection/pandemic-e-lit. Accessed 14 March 2024.

4. Here is the list of questions that structured the interviews:

    1. Can you describe your work in the exhibition and what inspired you to produce it?
    2. In most of the works in the exhibition, there is a sense that artists are trying to process and make sense of the pandemic situation through their work. Can you describe your artistic, literary and intellectual strategy for dealing with this?
    3. Can you say something about the genre or type of project you were drawn to creating during the pandemic or why it made sense to create in this particular form now?
    4. How do you think our cultural and intellectual consideration or understanding of the pandemic has shifted over the past year? Have any of the changes to our cultural life been positive or worth carrying on after the pandemic?
    5. Electronic Literature and digital art have always been mediated, online experiences. During this period virtually all of cultural life moved online. Did this mass migration online change the way you think about producing your work?
    6. Do you think that the audience reception and appreciation of e-lit has changed during this period?
    7. It has been argued that digital culture changed significantly from the open internet of the 1990s and early 2000s to a platform-based internet today that centres on social media, streaming platforms and mobile apps. Has this shift influenced your work?
    8. How has the pandemic changed your sense of your artistic community and social environment, in both positive and negative ways?
    9. The pandemic has come at a time of other larger crises, such the persistent climate crises and a cultural reckoning with racism. Are these other crises reflected in any way in your work?
    10. The pandemic affected everyone in ways that involved restrictions on our physical movements and environments. How did this localization in a specific place – culturally, geographically – affect your use of digital tools and response to the pandemic?
    11. What do you miss most about your life before the pandemic and what will you miss about your current life after the pandemic?

5. In Roskilde, the film was featured in an exhibition titled *Authors in Quarantine* which also used material from the *Covid E-lit – Digital Art from the Pandemic* exhibition in June 2021. The British Library has acquired it for their collection, where it will be available for viewing.
6. See for example the project 'Art in Quarantine' by Wreading Digits, http://art-in-quarantine.wreading-digits.com/ (Marques and Gago 2021, accessed 14 March 2024).
7. One of the initiatives focusing on the commemoration of the victims of the COVID-19 pandemic is Marked by Covid, relying on excavating individual stories and sharing private archives of survivors. Currently, a project to commemorate COVID-19 with an AR installation is underway (based on my conversation with Sarah Senk, one of the Marked by

Covid directors, at the MLA Convention 2023 in January 2023 in San Francisco) (Anna Nacher). Cf. Marked by Covid, https://www.markedbycovid.com; S. Senk, COVID-19 Memorials: Aesthetics and Politics, presentation at the MLA Convention 2023, 7 January 2023, San Francisco (conference presentation). A similar, Europe-based initiative is also available: The Covid-19 Visual Project, https://covid19visualproject.org/en/. Accessed 21 April 2023.

8. Kracauer writes: 'Everyone does his or her task on the conveyor belt, performing a partial function without grasping the totality. Like the pattern in the stadium, the organization stands above the masses, a monstrous figure whose creator withdraws it from the eyes of its bearers, and barely even observes it himself' (1995: 78).

9. Other works from our exhibition that work with algorithmic generative narrators should be mentioned and included here as well, e.g. Claire Fitch' *Ear for Surge*, and Amaranth Borsuk's *Curt Curtal Sonnet Corona*. Furthermore, the daily journal or chronicle is clearly part of the poetics of several works such as the ones of Xtine Burroughs, the Marino family, Bilal Mohammed and Sharon Daniel/Erik Loyer.

REFERENCES

Abrahams, Annie (2021), Zoom interview with Anna Nacher, Søren Bro Pold, Scott Rettberg & Ashleigh Steele, 21 March.

Andersen, Christian Ulrik and Pold, Søren (2018), *The Metainterface: The Art of Platforms, Cities and Clouds*, Cambridge, MA: MIT Press.

Beiguelman, Giselle (2021), Zoom interview with Anna Nacher, Søren Bro Pold, Scott Rettberg & Ashleigh Steele, 22 March.

Benjamin, Walter (1999), 'Little history of photography', in M. W. Jennings, H. Eiland and G. Smith (eds), *Selected Writings*, vol. 2, p. 2, Cambridge, MA: Belknap Press.

Burrough, Xtine (2021), Zoom interview with Anna Nacher, Søren Bro Pold, Scott Rettberg & Ashleigh Steele, 8 March.

Carla-Rossi, Giulia (2021), Zoom interview with Anna Nacher, Søren Bro Pold, Scott Rettberg & Ashleigh Steele, 14 March.

Daniel, Sharon and Loyer, Erik (2021), Zoom interview with Anna Nacher, Søren Bro Pold, Scott Rettberg & Ashleigh Steele, 22 March.

Erll, Astrid (2020a), 'Afterword: Memory worlds in times of Corona', *Memory Studies*, 13:5, pp. 861–74, https://doi.org/10.1177/1750698020943014.

Erll, Astrid (2020b), 'Will Covid-19 become part of collective memory', in M. Gerlof and R. Rittgerodt (eds), *13 Perspectives on the Pandemic Thinking in a State of Exception*, Berlin: Walter de Gruyter, pp. 45–50. https://blog.degruyter.com/wp-content/uploads/2021/02/DG_13perspectives_humanities.pdf. Accessed 19 March 2023.

Gillespie, Tarleton (2010), 'The politics of "platforms"', *New Media & Society*, 12:3, pp. 347–64, https://doi.org/10.1177/1461444809342738.

Grosser, Ben (2021a), 'On reading and being read in the pandemic: Software, interface, and The Endless Doomscroller', *Electronic Book Review*, 6 March 2022, https://doi.org/10.7273/7smg-bz36.

Grosser, Ben (2021b), Zoom interview with Anna Nacher, Søren Bro Pold, Scott Rettberg & Ashleigh Steele, 21 March.

Hayles, N. Katherine (2021), 'Novel Corona: Posthuman virus', *Critical Inquiry*, 47:S2, pp. S68–S72, https://doi.org/10.1086/711439.

Kracauer, Siegfried (1995), *The Mass Ornament* (trans. T. Y. Levin), Cambridge, MA: Harvard University Press.

Leavy, Patricia and Brinkmann, Svend (2014), 'Unstructured and semi-structured interviewing', in P. Leavy (ed.), *The Oxford Handbook of Qualitative Research*, Oxford: Oxford University Press, pp. 276–99, https://doi.org/10.1093/oxfordhb/9780199811755.013.030.

Lynteris, Christos (2019), *Human Extinction and Pandemic Imaginary*, London and New York: Routledge.

Marked by Covid, https://www.markedbycovid.com. Accessed 21 April 2023.

Marino, Mark and family (2021), Zoom interview with Anna Nacher, Søren Bro Pold, Scott Rettberg & Ashleigh Steele, 16 March.

Markham, Annette N., Harris, Anne and Luka, Mary Elizabeth (2020), 'Massive and microscopic sensemaking during Covid-19 times', *Qualitative Inquiry*, 27:7, pp. 759–66, https://doi.org/10.1177/1077800420962477.

Marques, Diogo and Gago, Ana (2021), 'Language |h|as a virus: From figure of thought to experimental laboratory'. *Platform (Post?) Pandemic – Electronic Literature Organization 2021 Conference and Festival*, Aarhus University, 24–28 May, https://conferences.au.dk/fileadmin/conferences/2021/ELO2021/Full_papers/Diogo_Marques_and_Ana_Gago_Language__H_as_a_Virus__from_figure_of_thought_to_experimental_laboratory__168.pdf. Accessed 19 March 2023.

Mohammed, Bilal (2021), Zoom interview with Anna Nacher, Søren Bro Pold, Scott Rettberg & Ashleigh Steele, 8 March.

Mooallem, Jon (2023), 'What happened to us', *The New York Times Magazine*, 22 February, https://www.nytimes.com/interactive/2023/02/22/magazine/covid-pandemic-oral-history.html?te=1&nl=the-new-york-times-magazine&emc=edit_ma_20230224. Accessed 21 April 2023.

Morrisey, Judd, Avnisan, Abraham and Jeffery, Mark (2021), Zoom interview with Anna Nacher, Søren Bro Pold, Scott Rettberg & Ashleigh Steele, 10 April.

Morton, Timothy (2013), 'Poisoned ground: Art and philosophy in the time of hyperobjects', *symploke*, 21:1, pp. 37–50, https://muse.jhu.edu/article/532809. Accessed 19 March 2023.

Nacher, Anna (2021), 'Afterword: As we may enact', in A. Klobucar (ed.), *The Community and the Algorithm: A Digital Interactive Poetics*, Wilmington, DE: Vernon Press, 155–64.

Nacher, Anna, Pold, Søren Bro, Rettberg, Scott and Steele, Ashleigh (2022), *Covid E-lit – Digital Art During the Pandemic*, https://retts.net/covid_elit/. Accessed 11 April 2023.

Nossiter, Adam (2020), 'Atget's Paris, 100 years later', *The New York Times*, 27 May, https://www.nytimes.com/2020/05/27/world/europe/paris-atget-coronavirus.html. Accessed 19 March 2023.

Piringer, Jörg (2021), Zoom interview with Anna Nacher, Søren Bro Pold, Scott Rettberg & Ashleigh Steele, 9 April.

Rettberg, Scott (2019), *Electronic Literature*, Oxford: Polity Press.

Saum-Pascual, Alex (2021), Zoom interview with Anna Nacher, Søren Bro Pold, Scott Rettberg & Ashleigh Steele, 7 March.

Senk, Sarah (2023), 'COVID-19 Memorials: Aesthetics and Politics', *Presentation at the MLA Convention 2023*, 7 January, San Francisco.

Singh, Juliette (2017), *Unthinking Mastery: Humanism and Decolonial Entanglements*, Durham: Duke University Press.

Taussig, Michael (2021), 'Would a Shaman help?' *Critical Inquiry*, 47:S2, pp. S33–S36, https://doi.org/10.1086/711430.

The Covid-19 Visual Project, https://covid19visualproject.org/en/. Accessed 21 April 2023.

Zellen, Jody (2021), Zoom interview with Anna Nacher, Søren Bro Pold, Scott Rettberg & Ashleigh Steele, 8 March.

13

Repetition and Revision: *The Plague*, 'St James' and the Humanities in Times of Crisis

Tony Whyton

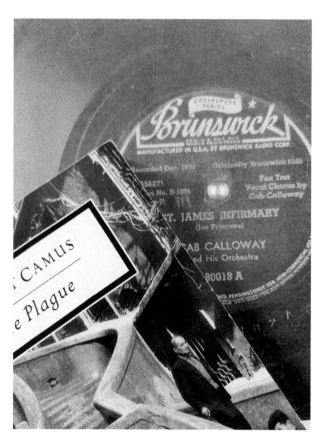

FIGURE 13.1: Albert Camus' *The Plague* and Cab Calloway's 'St James Infirmary'. Photo: Tony Whyton.

> From now on it can be said that plague was the concern of all of us. Hitherto, surprised as he may have been by the strange things happening around him, each individual citizen had gone about his business as usual, so far as this was possible. And no doubt he would have continued doing so. But once the town gates were shut, every one of us realized that all, the narrator included, were, so to speak, in the same boat, and each would have to adapt himself to the new conditions of life. Thus, for example, a feeling normally as individual as the ache of separation from those one loves suddenly became a feeling in which all shared alike and – together with fear – the greatest affliction of the long period of exile that lay ahead.
>
> (Camus 1989: 57)

Albert Camus' 1947 novel *La Peste* (translated to English in 1948 as *The Plague*) increased in sales during the COVID-19 pandemic, as readers searched for ways of understanding and engaging with pandemic times (Flood 2020). This interest also filtered into broader humanities research where literary scholars, historians, and philosophers began to examine ways in which the novel could help us to understand current social divisions and cultural crises (see, for example, Illing 2020; Jenkinson 2020; Meagher 2021; Sharpe 2020; Weiser 2023). *The Plague* is a novel that charts the fictional onset of bubonic plague in the French Algerian port city of Oran. The story depicts the gradual destruction of everyday life alongside an array of human responses displayed when people are held captive in a town riddled with infectious diseases. Told through the lens of the physician Dr Bernard Rieux, the narrative examines numerous relationships and encounters as plague grips the city, and explores many aspects of the human condition, from resilience to corruption, from religious fervour to the feeling of panic and despair. As a fictional narrative, Camus' text has been interpreted in several ways. On a literal level, the novel provides a fictional account of plague and its impact on humanity. On a symbolic level, the story has been interpreted as an allegory of the Nazi occupation of France in the Second World War. Equally, the text has been used to explore Camus' particular interpretation of the Absurd and his rejection of God (Foley 2008); it could read as a critique of French colonialism (Carroll 2008), or regarded structurally as a form of Greek tragedy, as we know in advance that there will be a horrible fate in store for many characters.

As a work of fiction, one of the enduring qualities of the novel is its versatility and malleability. *The Plague* works on many interpretative levels that can enable readers to relate the content of the story to their everyday lives and experiences. The novel provides a compelling way of exploring the emotions and responses to quarantine (or lockdown), the random nature of infection, and the threats to human existence during pandemic times. As the story unfolds, the gradual overwhelming of Oran is charted not only by the distress of the rise in daily deaths, the unpredictable nature of infection and the restriction of the movement of people but also by the way in which Camus provides a sense of the stifling of humanity, of personal freedoms and encounters, conveyed most clearly through the near absence of references to arts and culture. Indeed, one of the most shocking scenes in the novel is the public spectacle of an opera singer collapsing on stage during a performance of Gluck's *Orpheus*. Whilst at first seeming calm, panic ensues as the audience stampede for the exit, desperate to be free from potential infection. The destruction of the arts and the almost total absence of cultural references, activities, and events, works as a strategy to remind the reader of the precarity of life in plague times. This point is reinforced at the end of the novel when, post-plague, festivities, dance and celebrations return to the city as a mark of the new normal, humanity restored. Within the novel, whilst Camus makes seldom reference to arts and culture, somewhat unusually within the text, the story draws on two separate references to a recording of 'St James Infirmary', a blues song that remained popular throughout the twentieth century. 'St James Infirmary' is first heard within the setting of a hotel bar where Dr Rieux and Jean Tarrou (a character who will become the last victim of plague within the novel) attempt to persuade the journalist Raymond Rambert not to try to escape the city illegally. Rambert is a feature writer for a Paris newspaper who was visiting the city temporarily before the city was put under quarantine. Within the story, Rambert is desperate to leave, feeling unjustly exiled in a city in lockdown and he has attempted to plead to the authorities for his release without any success. Within the bar setting, conversations are 'half drowned by the stridence of *St. James Infirmary* coming from the loud-speaker just above their heads' (Camus 1989: 129). The second playing of 'St James Infirmary' takes place back in Rambert's apartment, where the conversation continues between Rieux, Rambert and Tarrou:

> 'So you haven't understood yet?' Rambert shrugged his shoulders almost scornfully.
> 'Understood what?'
> 'The plague.'
> 'Ah!' Rieux exclaimed.
> 'No, you haven't understood that it means exactly that – the same thing over and over again.'
> He went to the corner of the room and started a small gramophone.
> 'What's that record?' Tarrou asked. 'I've heard it before.'
> 'It's "St. James' Infirmary".'
> While the gramophone was playing, two shots rang out in the distance.
> 'A dog or a get-away,' Tarrou remarked.
> When, some moments later, the record ended, an ambulance bell could be heard clanging past under the window and receding into silence.

'Rather a boring record', Rambert remarked. 'And this must be the tenth time I've put it on today.'

'Are you really so fond of it?'

'No, but it's the only one I have'. And after a moment he added: 'That's what I said "it" was – the same thing over and over again.'

(Camus 1989: 134–35)

Reminiscent of Sartre's use of the recording of the song 'Some of These Days' in the 1938 novel *Nausea*, Camus serves to mirror the narrative events of *The Plague* with a musical reference that both echoes and embellishes the central themes of the story. Within the context of *The Plague*, 'St James Infirmary' not only provides a suitable death-themed sonic dimension to the ensuing crisis (indeed, as a blues, 'St James Infirmary' would have provided the soundtrack to many a New Orleans funeral, and would certainly have been heard during the time of the 1918 Influenza pandemic) but Camus also attempts to align the mechanical reproduction of the recording with the repetition of everyday life within a plague town. Here, Camus also mirrors Sartre's presentation of recordings as out of keeping with the experience of live music at the moment. In writing about the use of 'Some of These Days' in *Nausea*, for example, Paul Long suggests that Sartre 'expresses an abiding conceit that recordings are a secondary experience in popular and other kinds of musical practice' (Long 2019: 298). Within *The Plague*, the repetitious nature of 'St James Infirmary' is certainly presented as a negative aspect of recorded music. However, whether intended or not, the inclusion of 'St James Infirmary' also takes the reading of *The Plague* to a number of different levels. As with Long's discussion of 'Some of These Days' in *Nausea*, the specific recorded version of 'St James Infirmary' is not referenced within the text and this opens up the reader to ponder which version of the music is being played within the story. Here, as readers, our knowledge of the history of popular music intersects with the fictional world of *The Plague*, as 'St James Infirmary' had proven to be a hugely successful popular blues song recorded by numerous artists including Louis Armstrong, Sidney Bechet and Cab Calloway between 1928 and the publication of *The Plague* in 1947. Indeed, Calloway's 1933 version of the song had also been featured as part of the 1933 animated short, *Betty Boop in Snow White*.

Whilst the characters within *The Plague* bemoan the repetitive nature of the music, the context within which the recording is played and re-played within the novel is significant. The first encounter with the recording is within the public space of a hotel bar, whereas the second is within the private domain of Rambert's apartment. The change in context also anticipates the increase in intensity within the novel, as the impact of the plague on peoples' lives leads to changes in behaviour and a gradual move from the public to the private sphere, from freedom of movement to incarceration. Equally, the playing of music on record and the portability of this technology are suggestive of the way in which music can transport us to other spaces. Recordings are not read the same every time we hear them and can ignite our imagination; they have the capacity to transform our lives even when we are in a state of confinement.

The choice of 'St James Infirmary' is perhaps suggestive of a narrative self-awareness on behalf of Camus not only in relation to the theme of the song itself but also in terms of the ambiguity of the musicians the central characters are listening to within the different scenes. As a popular song, 'St James Infirmary' emerged through numerous former lives and versions, borrowings and adaptations. Indeed, the song itself seems to embody the notion of repetition and revision, said to be one of the hallmarks of African American arts and the aesthetic of the blues (Gates 1988; Murray 1989). The absence of a specific reference to a particular version of 'St James Infirmary' encourages us to think about the problem of provenance of the song, the different versions that have existed through time, and the way in which the music itself has proliferated in different cultures and settings, including fictional places. Indeed, there are several sources devoted to charting the supposed origins of 'St James Infirmary' itself; from that claim, it links to a range of English and Celtic Folk songs, to other blues forms and popular songs, to a link with a folk song that was documented in the Appalachians in 1918 (Harwood 2022). Consider Robert W. Harwood's *I Went Down to 'St James Infirmary'* (2022), a book that seeks to unravel and engage with the song and what is, at times, a speculative journey of creation. Harwood draws on the work of the English folklorist A. L. Lloyd to explain how some popular songs emerge through forms of musical, lyrical and geographical migration. In a folk tradition, for example, Lloyd describes the way in which a song may be devised by a farmer in the field and would later pass this on to others in a pub. Following the performance, the song may be recounted but also misremembered and this leads to a chain of repetition and revision. Quoting Lloyd, Harwood continues the hypothetical journey of the song:

> 'Perhaps a carter carries it into the next county and introduces it to a new community. The song spreads from mouth to mouth, place-to-place, parent to child, age to age, and so enters the vast reservoir of collective memory. There it will lead a capricious life of fluctuating fortune. It may divide into countless variants, some close to the original, some so far-removed as to constitute virtually new songs'. It might temporarily or permanently disappear, 'no longer corresponding to the psychological need of the time. Perhaps other variants more in tune with the spirit of the era may chase the "original" right out of the folklore circuit'. Eventually [...] a single version might become dominant, and hold sway for many years.
>
> (Harwood 2022: 39)

Interestingly, if you read the above quotation again and substitute the word 'song' for 'virus', the passage could easily be read as a common description of the recent spread of COVID-19. Like a virus itself, 'St James Infirmary' manifests itself as a variant, a distant relation to other forms. There may be some resemblances to other songs but it is a new entity in itself, finding meaning for present-day listeners. This point is echoed in Jennifer Cooke's work (2009), which explores post-outbreak plague representations across a range of cultural discourses, including literature, drama, psychoanalysis, political rhetoric and film. Cooke examines the way in which plagues throughout history have generated creative responses in the arts and examines how the legacies of plague can be seen in different forms of representation. For Cooke, creative representations of the plague such as Camus' *The Plague*

> reveal the fragility of the social bond, the fascination of diseased spectacle and the literal and metaphorical power of pestilence. They highlight, too, the way in which structures of ritual surrounding the contagious and the taboo, while they may have been practically supplanted, are still operative under new guises in discourse.
> (Cooke 2009: 14)

Cooke suggests that the legacies of these creative representations function in a similar way to the plague itself; art, literature, music and film all have 'disseminative properties and they spread contagiously [...] throughout different discourses and art forms, with little regard for the boundaries which might ordinarily separate domains' (Cooke 2009: 14).

The array of meanings and interpretations linked to the novel is representative of the fact that 'Camus had always advocated multireferentiality, that is, multiple readings of "the plague"' (Weiser 2023: 19). Whether Camus is commenting on events in history, such as the Nazi occupation of France, the real historical presence of plague in cities such as Oran, or is conjuring up a link to experiences of time and sound at the moment with references to popular music on record, the experience of *The Plague* is immediately an intertextual one. Alongside multiple interpretations of the text, the intertextual relationship between *The Plague* and 'St James's Infirmary' also illustrates how cultural objects can form a dialectical relationship with one another. Considering the provenance and journey of the recording of 'St James Infirmary', we can re-read Camus and think differently about the novel, the role of popular music in different historical settings, and of the sound world of a particular place in literature, albeit a place that blends imaginative fiction with references to the real world.

These readings, re-readings, comparisons and creative responses say not only much about the power of literature but also of the humanities more broadly; not only in the way in which the humanities encourage us to learn from the past – the repetition and revision seen in the pages of literature and the sounds of music – but also in the power of writing to engage with human emotion and to convey experiences of everyday life. In discussing the impact of *The Plague*, Peg Brand Weiser stresses that, in many ways, the novel represents a triumph of fiction over facts which, in a different sense, could be seen as a neat way of demonstrating the value of the humanities in dealing with real-world problems, the power of qualitative approaches over quantitative methods. Instead of focusing purely on the presentation of data and numbers, such as the listing of daily death rates or the presentation of statistical surveys, *The Plague* presents us with 'an account of people thrown together by fate who succeed in pulling together, acting in solidarity, and surviving the worst conditions of the plague' (Weiser 2023: 6). Weiser argues that writing an account of plague could have easily resulted in a limited, documentary-style work of nonfiction or a dry philosophical text. Instead, Camus demonstrates how story-telling can be more valuable to people than simple facts in times of crisis:

> Strategically, Camus chose fiction to convey facts. *The Plague* is not just fiction, since it is based on haunting facts from the historical past; nor is it merely literary journalism, as it attends to newsworthy details of everyday life in a storytelling setting. It may function as escape fiction, but our escape is illusory as we ourselves – living in a pandemic reproducing the restrictive conditions like those of bubonic plague in 1940s Oran – identify with the actions of fictional characters like those we witness in real life: in the media, on the streets, in hospitals, on Zoom, within our own families. Our lived experiences – the starting point for phenomenologists seeking to chart the theoretical – map onto Camus's narrative, confirming Simone de Beauvoir's similar intuition to choose to write fiction over philosophy.
> (Weiser 2023: 20)

From this, novels such as *The Plague* also highlight the importance of the arts and humanities – and of culture more broadly – in contributing to meaning making, our sense of being, belonging and understanding in the world. Through the creativity of the novel and its intertextual threads, we can be encouraged to think about our relationship to history, to each other, and of the precarity of the human condition more broadly. Unlike the central characters in *The Plague*, we can move beyond the simple assumption that things simply repeat to explore ways in which contexts change, meanings are revised, and differences occur in terms of the spread and impact of plague. We can also consider how the technologies of a particular age can serve to either combat or contribute to the spread of disease, be it new technologies that lead to breakthroughs in the development of vaccines or the fact that, tangentially, for example, air travel serves to facilitate the rapid global spread of viruses.

Despite the end of the plague ending with a return to some form of normality and festivities, Dr Rieux's final words provide a word of caution, reminding us both of the cyclical nature of plague and also of humanity's ignorance in learning from the past:

> [A]s he listened to the cries of joy rising from the town, Rieux remembered that such joy is always imperilled. He knew what those jubilant crowds did not know but could have learned from books: that the plague bacillus never dies or disappears for good; that it can lie dormant for years and years in furniture and linen-chests; that it bides its time in bedrooms, cellars, trunks, and bookshelves; and that perhaps the day would come when, for the bane and the enlightening of men, it would rouse up its rats again and send them forth to die in a happy city.
>
> (Camus 1989: 252)

This closing statement provides us with the sobering thought that crises are an inevitable part of the human condition. It also reminds us that we should not neglect the humanities. As Dr Rieux's words suggest, if we remain ignorant of education and do not learn from the past (from the books he describes), then we remain ill-prepared to deal with the inevitable crises of the future. As an indication of the relevance of *The Plague* to current crises, we can not only see the direct relationship between COVID-19 and recent experiences of the global pandemic within the narrative but also the allegorical qualities of the book, of occupation, displacement and trauma, which also seem as relevant today as they did in 1947. I am currently writing this chapter less than 250 km from the Ukrainian border, a year after the Russian invasion. Over the past year, I've seen streams of people pouring out of trains, seeking refuge, traumatized by the effects of war. Within this context, I cannot avoid thinking about the interrelationship between plague and war and the ways in which the neglect of the humanities has contributed to the spread of misinformation, the presentation of skewed histories, and a lack of public discourse around the past and its relationship to the present. Watching television accounts and following social media, it becomes increasingly difficult to identify concepts of truth and justice when there is limited contextual knowledge in circulation or clear examples of critical thinking within the public sphere. This collection is a clarion call for the humanities to play a more central role in finding an answer to everyday crises and global challenges, be it plague, war or appropriate responses to environmental change. The humanities can provide an understanding of the nature of crises, drawing attention to rarely perceived links between past and present, in order to work towards a more sustainable model for the future. The humanities build bridges, and they are key to finding empathy with others through the promotion of dialogue to encourage historical and cultural understanding. The humanities can develop a tolerance and respect for cultural differences, educating and engaging with communities so that responses to future crises are more effective, coordinated and timely. As Camus' *The Plague* and the contributions set out in this collection demonstrate, the humanities have the ability to engage with the complexities of human life, the behavioural patterns and rituals that create a sense of order and tie into different values and belief systems. As the examples within this collection have demonstrated, the humanities can decipher media communications, identify underlying ideologies and draw on examples from history and different cultural contexts to illuminate the present. Times of plague inevitably trigger creative responses, whether it is finding new ways of working or adapting to change, or creating new art as an affirmation of living, and exploring what it is to be human. Within this world, we can learn from the past, document human experience, encourage dialogue and cultural understanding, and imagine a different future. Repetition and revision; this is the power of the humanities.

REFERENCES

Camus, Albert (1989), *The Plague* (trans. Stuart Gilbert), New York & London: Penguin.

Carroll, David (2008), *Albert Camus the Algerian: Colonialism, Terrorism, Justice*, New York: Columbia University Press.

Cooke, Jennifer Cooke (2009), *Legacies of Plague in Literature, Theory and Film*, London: Palgrave MacMillan.

Flood, Alison (2020), 'Publishers report sales boom in novels about fictional epidemics', *The Guardian*, 5 March, https://www.theguardian.com/books/2020/mar/05/publishers-report-sales-boom-in-novels-about-fictional-epidemics-camus-the-plague-dean-koontz. Accessed 20 May 2023.

Foley, John (2008), *Albert Camus: From the Absurd to Revolt*, New York: Routledge.

Gates, Henry Louis, Jr. (1988), *The Signifying Monkey: A Theory of African-American Literary Criticism*, New York: Oxford University Press.

Harwood, Robert W. (2022), *I Went Down to 'St James Infirmary'*, Los Angeles, CA: Genius Music Books.

Illing, Sean (2020), 'This is a time for solidarity; What Albert Camus's "The Plague" can teach us about life in a pandemic', *Vox*, 15 March, https://www.vox.com/2020/3/13/21172237/coronavirus-covid-19-albert-camus-the-plague. Accessed 20 May 2023.

Jenkinson, Clay S. (2020), 'Why we should be reading Albert Camus during the pandemic', *Governing*, 26 May, https://www.governing.com/context/Why-We-Should-Be-Reading-Albert-Camus-During-the-Pandemic.html. Accessed 20 May 2023.

Long, Paul (2019), 'The poetics of recorded time: Listening again to popular music history', *Popular Music History*, 12:3, pp. 295–315.

Meagher, Robert E. (2021), *Albert Camus and the Human Crisis*, New York & London: Pegasus Books.

Murray, Albert (1989), *Stompin' the Blues*, New York: Da Capo Press.

Sharpe, Matthew (2020), 'Guide to the classics: Albert Camus "The Plague"', *The Conversation*, 6 April, https://theconversation.com/guide-to-the-classics-albert-camus-the-plague-134244. Accessed 21 May 2023.

Weiser, Peg Brand (ed.) (2023), *Camus' The Plague: Philosophical Perspectives*, New York: Oxford University Press.

CONCLUSION

14

The Power of the Humanities

Wojciech Sowa

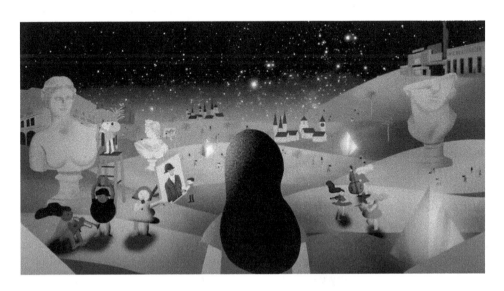

FIGURE 14.1: A screenshot from Annlin Chao's animation *Humanities Matter* (2020).

At the beginning of this collection, we started our journey in the distant past with an illustration of a cuneiform fragment of a Hittite prayer, pleading gods to end the plague. Travelling through time, through languages and cultures, we could see the same anxiety and distress manifesting in human behaviour in such a critical moment as a pandemic (cf. Sofaer in Chapter 2). With this volume, we wanted to highlight the significance of history, language, narrative, culture, ethics and other domains of humanities research in understanding the impact of the pandemic, not only in the short term but in the future by providing a longer perspective on changes brought about by the crisis, in conjunction with research in the natural, life and social sciences. How will the history of COVID be told or written down? Is this pandemic different from the previous episodes from Antiquity (as discussed by Steger in Chapter 6), the medieval and early modern periods right up to the recent times in the way diseases were spread and were fought, documented, represented and remembered or even erased from public memory?

It seems that encountering the plague from the perspective of humanities must include, next to the various kinds of responses (media, political or legal, cf. Baranowska and Gliszczynska-Grabias in Chapter 4 for the perspective of the human rights), also the emphasis on the language and rhetoric of the disease and the diverse narratives created by it, as these yield a mirror of ourselves and our societies. Here one has to underline the role of literature, which is a peculiar but powerful tool for cognition. By telling a fictional story, it allows us to see and understand general, as real as possible, patterns of human behaviour.

The sensory and affective realms of experience charted in literary texts are a crucial component of the cultural history of contagious diseases. The field of literary criticism, for example, has long been attentive to the nuances of narrative representations of health crises, pestilences and diseases more broadly. The current COVID-19 emergency has thrown into sharp relief the need to gain a better understanding of how humanity has learned to cope with collective calamities and with the very notion of contagion. The literary texts (except for the historical value) inform us about the socially destructive effects of the disease, e.g. alienation, which is experienced by people living in fear of the virus, and the defence mechanisms caused by it, increased distrust and stigmatization of strangers, susceptibility to conspiracy theories and the scapegoat mechanism. Whether it is an allegorical historical novel set in fifteenth-century Brabant (as Szczypiorski 1971) or a quoted Plague Prayer by Mursilis II, the problem of 'Who's to blame' remains the same; in many cases, it is left unanswered or the one to blame is the foreigner, the Other. And this, as we learn from history, leads to outbreaks of various forms of civil disobedience, and in many cases, it may lead also to various forms of organized violence, even war.

This is exactly where the intellectual power of the humanities manifests, as the entire domain seems to be involved with the COVID crisis. It seems to prompt individuals and societies to reflect on the mortality, and the fragility of the human condition, which has led to increased interest in philosophical and existential questions related to life, death and the general purpose of our being (see Roszak-Orlowski in Chapter 3 with an interesting observation on the ritualization of the medical means to fight the plague in the current COVID crisis in the Roman Catholic church). The historical research investigates the societal and political implications of the plague – the impact on healthcare systems, the social and economic disparities or the political response at the governmental level contributing to our understanding of how societies generally respond to global crises and shape future policies (cf. two contributions in this context by Brown-Robillaird in Chapter 7 and Giry-Deloison in Chapter 5).

The pandemic has raised ethical questions regarding public health policies, resource allocation and individual liberties, and what is the balance between public safety and personal freedom. The ethics of vaccine distribution and the responsibilities of governments and individuals during a health crisis impose the question of individual responsibilities towards others.

Interesting is the linguistic phenomenon, as the pandemic has introduced new vocabulary and terminology related to COVID-19, public health measures, and vaccines. Linguists and communication scholars analyse the language used in public health messaging, media coverage and online discourse to understand how information is created, circulated interpreted and sometimes misinterpreted (see Majewska on the impact of the pandemics on language in Chapter 9 and Petrauskaitė-Amilevičius on the intimidating use of the language in the COVID context in Chapter 10).

With physical distancing measures in place, there has been a significant shift towards digital platforms for cultural and artistic experiences. The digital humanities have gained prominence, with museums, libraries and cultural institutions offering virtual exhibitions, online lectures and digital archives. This has expanded access to cultural resources and facilitated new forms of engagement with the humanities, which before had the tendency to hide in the Ivory Tower. It has also been a great challenge for the educational sphere in order to assure the continuity and inclusivity of the process (cf. the contributions by Brandallero in Chapter 11 and Nacher-Bro Pold-Rettberg in Chapter 12).

It seems that the notion of culture has been reinterpreted. As with every epidemic also, COVID-19 has inspired many authors and artists to explore and express their experiences and emotions during these times. Literature and creative arts have served as a medium for people to process their thoughts and feelings, providing solace and fostering a sense of shared understanding. The culture being felt by many as a mere 'entertainment' (without distinction into a 'simple' and more 'sophisticated'), it gradually evolved into a joint creative endeavour, an experiment and improvisation on a scale not known before. It appeared that even when physically closed and isolated in our homes we strive to meet others, and do creative things together. In this respect, the interplay between the various forms of cultural activities and the public spaces, whether material, symbolic or virtual became a scene for a range of new responses to such challenges, e.g. globalization, digitization or migration.

The power of the humanities lies in their ability to deepen our understanding of the human experience, stimulate critical thinking and foster empathy and cultural appreciation. By exploring the realms of literature, philosophy, history, art and music, we engage with the ideas and creations that define us as human beings. In a world driven by rapid technological advancements, the humanities remind us of our shared humanity and serve as a beacon of insight, compassion and enlightenment. They are not merely an academic pursuit but an essential part of our intellectual and emotional growth, empowering us to create a more inclusive, empathetic and harmonious society.

More than ever the humanities play a special role today. In a time of fundamental debates about the nature of Europe and the European project, including more and more the emphasized word 'crisis', the humanities allow us to understand more comprehensively what Europe is, what it has been in the past, and what its future options may be. The humanities have provided us with invaluable tools to navigate the complexities of the COVID-19 pandemic and have equipped us with the intellectual and emotional resilience needed to confront and adapt to the challenges brought about by the pandemic.

In the previous chapter, Whyton explored the allegorical use of plague in Albert Camus' *The Plague* as a symbol of the Nazi occupation of France. The unexpected outbreak of the war in February 2022 in the reality, slowly recovering from the COVID-19 pandemic came as a shock, demonstrated the fragility of the political system and has shaken the fundaments of Europe's economic prosperity. It also showed the power of propaganda and manipulation to the scale not known before, spreading in the globalized world in a way resembling the virus. The conflict also saw the use of social media on an unprecedented scale as a form of a 'weapon'. This forced the international community to think again about the nature of information, the notion of truth, the ethics and the true reasons for this conflict. The crisis has revealed how important it is to understand the history of the region, the complicated relations between Russia and those territories it wrongly claims historically and culturally, the linguistic dimensions and religious dimensions of such claims to particular territories and why all these elements have been misused in the imperialistic discourse created by the Kremlin. In other words, we can't make much progress in thinking through this crisis without some depth of historical analysis of Putin and his ambitions (whatever the reasons they may have), and also without trying to understand the depth of the Ukrainian spirit and identity behind the resistance. As maybe some of us share the experience of feeling powerless while seeing the reports from the front line, asking ourselves what the point of our research is in such an environment, it seems that especially researchers in the humanities could play a significant role in providing valuable insights and contributing to the understanding of various aspects related to the conflict, for example by studying the historical and cultural context: to delve into the historical and cultural factors that have contributed to the outbreak of the war. This may involve examining Ukraine's complicated history, its delicate relationship with Russia and Poland and the dynamics of national identity within the country. Then also the humanities can examine narratives and memory surrounding the conflict, analysing how different groups involved in the conflict construct and propagate their own narratives, as well as how collective memory is shaped and is (has been) contested. One of the most important aspects is the humanitarian and human rights perspective, which involves examining the impact of the conflict on civilians, including issues such as displacement, access to healthcare and education, and violations of human rights. Raising awareness, advocating for justice and contributing to policy discussions regarding humanitarian interventions and the protection of human rights are also natural activities undertaken by the humanities.

All these presuppose engagement in interdisciplinary collaboration. Given the complex nature of the conflict, researchers in the humanities should strengthen collaborations with their peers from other disciplines. Interdisciplinary research can provide a more comprehensive understanding of the conflict and generate nuanced insights that can inform policy and decision-making, resulting in exploring theories and practices of peacebuilding and conflict resolution that may be applicable to this particular context.

The humanities are essential to this enquiry, and they are also best prepared to address such questions. Only the humanities may demonstrate clearly how different pasts are actively and instrumentally used, and to what ends, always in connection to past or present debates or transformations in Europe. They will examine which historically informed discourses and actions in society are promoted, mobilized and legitimized, and which mechanisms lie behind the work of historical understanding – in arts, film, literature, drama, media, landscapes, public spaces, languages, philosophy and religions as well as in research, education, politics, economics and journalism. This knowledge will enable us to see more clearly the complex ways in which our cultural diversity has been formed, and the dynamics by which it may be shaped and directed in the future. It will explore and systematize exactly what it means to be a 'reflective society', enabling us to better understand processes of historical development, innovation, and social change that are fundamental to the human condition.

The main topic of this volume, i.e. addressing 'the plague' from various perspectives of the humanities, in both 'traditional' and 'modern' ways, could demonstrate that the humanities can identify 'grand challenges' of their own. Typically, the ones that are cited in the discussion at the European level are Bio-Med or STEM-led, even where there are obvious 'human' dimensions (e.g. climate change/digital transformation). It seems, however, that it may require redefining what humanities really are, trying to divert from the typical disputes about which discipline is still part of the domain and which is not, and to focus instead on their main goals, which, according to the Humanities in the European Research Area (HERA) network, should be then a transformation of the social imaginary by making explicit the multitude of vocabularies used to describe general human experience.

As no vocabulary naturally prevails over any other, humanities should be understood not so much as a cluster of academic disciplines but rather as a critical disposition of mind that puts in crisis the ossified structures of thinking. Since this work is still dramatically needed in contemporary academia, the modernizing project of the humanities remains unfinished and must be further developed.

In today's world, we all have to do more to champion the humanities in everyday life: the R&D innovation-driven policies very often cannot accept proposed research ideas working with something 'immaterial', not 'target' oriented and thus felt as 'useless' by many, even though there are the humanities which make us aware of the relativity of what we do with the world. For this reason, they could take the place of basic science, because their subject matter is not 'this or that', this particular object or that (e.g. literature of the Victorian period, Cubist painting or passive voice or attributive), but actually human existence in its various more or less institutionalized forms.

Contributors

DARIUS AMILEVIČIUS is an associate professor at the Department of Informatics and Chief Researcher at the Interdisciplinary Digital Resources Driven Research Institute of VMU. He has 20 years of experience in research and teaching and has worked as an expert in the AI Think-Tank of the Ministry of Economics of Lithuania since 2017. Darius is a member of the Confederation of Laboratories for Artificial Intelligence Research in Europe (CLAIRE), an expert of the Research Council of Lithuania and a member of the European AI Alliance and CLARIN ERIC. His research interests cover artificial intelligence technologies and natural language technologies.

*****

GRAŻYNA BARANOWSKA is an assistant professor at the Institute of Law Studies of the Polish Academy of Sciences and Marie Skłodowska-Curie postdoctoral researcher at the Center for Fundamental Rights of the Hertie School. She did post-doctoral research at the consortium 'Memory Laws in European and Comparative Perspective' (MELA: 2016–19), and currently supports the research consortium: 'The Challenge of Populist Memory Politics for Europe: Towards Effective Responses to Militant Legislation on the Past' (MEMOCRACY, 2021–24). Since August 2022, she is also one of the five independent experts in the UN Working Group on Enforced and Involuntary Disappearances. Her research covers several topics in the areas of international human rights law and migration law, with a special focus on disappeared and missing persons, border violence and memory laws. In 2021, Intersentia published her first book on the *Rights of Families of Disappeared Persons*, while her articles appeared in journals such as the *Netherlands Quarterly of Human Rights*, *International Review of the Red Cross*, *Israel Law Review* and *European Convention on Human Rights Law Review*.

*****

SARA BRANDELLERO teaches and researches at Leiden University's Centre for the Arts in Society (LUCAS), where she specializes in the culture of Brazil and the globalized Portuguese-speaking world more broadly, including in transnational, postcolonial perspectives. Her research centres on questions of spatial practice and agency, cultural imaginaries of night-time, travel and diasporic narratives and migration and the relationship between culture, politics and democracy.

* * * * *

JAMES BROWN is the knowledge exchange programme manager at the University of Sheffield. He has a background in academic history, specializing in cultures of drinking and intoxication in early modern England, and was previously a research associate and project manager of the HERA-funded research project Intoxicating Spaces: The Impact of New Intoxicants on Urban Spaces in Europe, 1600–1850 (https://www.intoxicatingspaces.org/). He is also interested in the digital humanities; project and programme management; and public engagement, knowledge exchange and impact.

* * * * *

CHARLES GIRY-DELOISON is vice chair of the HERA Joint Research Programme Board and Emeritus Professor of early modern history at the University of Artois (Arras, France). Professor Giry-Deloison has extensively written on English foreign policy in the late fifteenth to early seventeenth century and on Anglo-French relations during that period.

* * * * *

ALEKSANDRA GLISZCZYŃSKA-GRABIAS is an assistant professor at the Institute of Law Studies of the Polish Academy of Sciences. She is an expert in the fields of anti-discrimination law, constitutional law, freedom of speech and memory laws and is co-editor and co-author of *Law and Memory: Towards Legal Governance of History* (CUP, 2017) and *Constitutionalism under Stress* (OUP, 2020). She was a Braudel Fellow at the European University Institute, Bohdan Winiarski Fellow at the Lauterpacht Centre of the University of Cambridge and Graduate Fellow at the Yale University Initiative for the Study of Antisemitism. Principal Investigator in international research consortiums: 'The Challenge of Populist Memory Politics for Europe: Towards Effective Responses to Militant Legislation on the Past' (MEMOCRACY, 2021–24) and 'Memory Laws in European and Comparative Perspective' (MELA: 2016–19).

* * * * *

AGNIESZKA JELEWSKA is a professor at the Adam Mickiewicz University in Poznań, Poland, Deputy Dean of the Department of Anthology and Cultural Studies, and director of the Humanities/Art/Technology Research Center AMU. She has served as a visiting fellow at Kent University, Canterbury, UK. She held lectures and workshops at Emerson College Boston, Folkwang Universität der Kunst, Essen and Mahindra Humanities Center at Harvard University. Jelewska has authored and co-edited the books *Ecotopias, The Expansion of Technoculture* (2013 in Polish), *Art and Technology in Poland, From Cybercommunism to the Culture of Makers* (2014), *Postcollectivity, Situated Knowledge and Practices* (2024, as co-editor with Michał Krawczak and Julian Reid), *Spectral Archives of Nuclear Gaia* (2025, co-authored with Michał Krawczak) and a number of articles. She examines the transdisciplinary relations between science, art, culture and technology in the twentieth and twenty-first centuries, their social and political dimension. She is also a curator and co-creator of art and science projects: Transnature is Here (2013); Post-Apocalypsis (2015) – awarded a golden medal from PQ 2016; Anaesthesia (2016); PostHuman Data (2019).

*****

MALGORZATA MAJEWSKA graduated in Polish philology at the Jagiellonian University. There she completed her Ph.D. in linguistic pragmatics on how people belittle themselves through words. Then her scientific interests turned to the media and since 2005 she has been working at the Institute of Journalism, Media and Social Communication of the Jagiellonian University. Her research interests focus on language seen from the perspective of cognitive linguistics. Majewska believes that linguistics places too much emphasis on linguistic correctness and normativity, and too little attention is paid to how people actually talk to each other and what image of the world they build. She argues that understanding these details of linguistic use, often treated as errors by language purists, is the key to understanding other people. Majewska wrote a book about the relationship between privacy and media and, at the same time, is strongly involved in promoting and popularizing linguistic knowledge. She recently published the book *I speak, therefore I am.*

*****

ANNA NACHER is an associate professor at the Institute of Audiovisual Arts and Faculty of Management and Social Communication at Jagiellonian University. Nacher is a 2020 Fulbright alumna and a member of the Board of Directors of the Electronic Literature Organization. Her research primarily centres around contemporary art, digital aesthetics and media, with a focus on new media art, electronic literature and sound art. She occasionally ventures into ecological humanities and postcolonial theory. She has published articles in journals (*European Journal of Women's Studies, Hyperrhiz, Electronic Book Review, Acoustic Space, Communications +1*) and contributed chapters to various edited volumes. In addition to her academic pursuits, Anna Nacher is also a musician and sound artist with a particular emphasis on voice and field recordings. Since 2021, she has been collaborating with Victoria Vesna on various projects, such as Alien Star Dust Online Meditation, Noise Aquarium Meditation and Breath Library. Beyond her professional accomplishments, she is an active member of permaculture community, which she has been building in the Carpathian mountains since 2014. For more information and a full list of publications, refer to http://breathlibrary.org

*****

PIOTR PAWEL ORŁOWSKI holds a Ph.D. in theology and is interested in business ethics, contemporary theory of leadership and the history of pilgrimage on the Camino de Santiago; is co-founder of the *Pro Futuro Theologiae* Foundation and a member of its Council; organizer of scientific exchange between Polish and Spanish universities; co-owner and President of the Management Board of Nova Trading and Nova Metale as well as shareholder and Chairman of the Supervisory Board of Nicrometal; organizer of scientific conferences in the field of Thomism; and coordinator of research projects on religious freedom. Among numerous professional activities and scientific research passions, he plays one more, the most important life role – the father of his six children, who give him satisfaction and motivation to take up further challenges.

*****

RŪTA PETRAUSKAITĖ is a habilitated doctor in linguistics since 2006 employed as a professor at Vytautas Magnus University. Presently she has the position of the director of the Institute of Digital Resources and Interdisciplinary Research. Her research interests comprise a range of topics from corpus and computational linguistics to discourse analyses. She has published six books and more than 90 research papers. Previously she was a Vice-President of the Research Council of Lithuania and the Chair of the Committee of Social Sciences and Humanities, also involved in the activities of the program committees for Social Sciences and Humanities at the European Science Foundation as well as at two EU Framework Programmes (FP7 and Horizon 2020), COST Scientific Committee, ERA NET PLUS network board of HERA (Humanities in the European Research Area),

Science Europe Research Data working group, the EOSC Governing Board, the ESFRI Forum and CLARIN ERIC research infrastructure.

* * * * *

SØREN BRO POLD, Ph.D., is an associate professor of digital Aesthetics. He publishes digital and media aesthetics and art, e.g. on interface criticism, software studies, platform culture, electronic literature, net art, software art, critical design and aesthetics in design, critical data studies and digital culture. He was part of the research project COVID-19 and Electronic Literature and is currently co-leader of the research program Cultures and Practices of Digital Technologies. Furthermore, he was chair of the Electronic Literature Organisation's conference Platform (Post?) Pandemic (2021).

* * * * *

SCOTT RETTBERG is the director of the Center for Digital Narrative, a Norwegian Center of Research Excellence. He is a professor of digital culture in the Department of Linguistic, Literary and Aesthetic Studies at the University of Bergen, Norway. Rettberg was the project leader of Electronic Literature as a Model of Creativity and Innovation in Practice (ELMCIP) from 2010 to 2013. Rettberg is the leader of the Bergen Electronic Literature Research Group and director of the ELMCIP Electronic Literature Knowledge Base. Rettberg is the author or co-author of novel-length works of electronic literature, combinatory poetry and films, including *The Unknown, Kind of Blue, Implementation, Frequency, The Catastrophe Trilogy, Three Rails Live, Toxi*City, Hearts and Minds: The Interrogations Project* and others. His creative work has been exhibited online and at art venues, including the Venice Biennale, Santa Monica Museum in Barcelona, the Inova Gallery, Rom 8, the Chemical Heritage Foundation Museum, Palazzo dell Arti Napoli, Beall Center, the Slought Foundation, The Krannert Art Museum and elsewhere. Rettberg is the co-founder and served as the first executive director of the nonprofit Electronic Literature Organization. Rettberg's book *Electronic Literature* (Polity 2018) is a foundational study of the history and genres of electronic literature and was the winner of the N. Katherine Hayles Award for Criticism of Electronic Literature.

* * * * *

GABRIELLE ROBILLIARD is a historian specializing in early modern medicine, intoxicants and food, as well as maritime and global history. Her publications focus on midwifery, medical consumption of intoxicants and coffeehouse sociability in early modern Germany. Gabrielle studied history and modern German literature in Melbourne, Berlin, Cambridge and Göttingen before completing her Ph.D. in history at the University of Warwick in 2011. She later worked as a postdoctoral researcher on the HERA-funded research project Intoxicating Spaces: The Impact of New Intoxicants on Urban Spaces in Europe, 1600–1850 (https://www.intoxicatingspaces.org/) and is currently a research associate of the Göttingen Academy-funded Prize Papers Project (https://www.prizepapers.de/) at Oldenburg University.

* * * * *

Piotr Roszak is a professor of theology at Nicolaus Copernicus University in Toruń, Poland; associated professor at the University of Navarra, Pamplona, Spain, where he obtained his Ph.D. in 2009. Member of the Pontifical Academy of St. Thomas Aquinas; Editor-in-Chief of the *Scientia et Fides* journal dedicated to science-religion debate, and director of the series *Scholastica Thoruniensia*, where the Polish translations of medieval biblical commentaries are published. Together with Mateusz Przanowski OP, he is leading the project of 'Opera Omnia' of St. Thomas Aquinas in Poland. He has obtained several grants from the Templeton Foundation, National Science Centre in Poland and in Spain. He is an honorary member of the Pontificia Academia Mariana Internationalis and the *Comite de Expertos del Camino de Santiago* in Spain. He recently published (together with Jörgen Vijgen): *Reading the Church Fathers with St. Thomas Aquinas Historical and Systematical Perspectives* (Brepols: Turnhout 2021).

* * * * *

Joanna Sofaer is a professor of archaeology at the University of Southampton, co-director of the Southampton Institute for Arts and Humanities (SIAH), Director of Archaeology for the Creative Industries, and was Humanities in the European Research Area (HERA) Knowledge Exchange and Impact Fellow (2017–23). Her current work focuses on the role of cultural assets in supporting health and wellbeing, working in partnership with communities, health professionals, the third sector and cultural organizations. She is PI for the UKRI-funded project Pathways to Health Through Cultures of Neighbourhoods and PI for Heritage and Wellbeing for NHS Staff (HerWellNHS) funded by Historic England in collaboration with Portsmouth Hospitals University NHS Trust. She works with the National Trust on the Heritage Perception and Wellbeing project and led Places of Joy: Heritage After Lockdown. Joanna is also interested in the past as inspiration for contemporary creative practice and creativity in prehistoric material culture.

She has led and partnered on several transnational European projects, including the HERA-funded project Creativity and Craft Production in Middle and Late Bronze Age Europe.

*****

WOJCIECH SOWA is chair of the HERA Joint Research Programme Board and professor at the Institute of Classical Philology, Jagiellonian University. Professor Sowa is an internationally-renowned scholar of Indo-European Linguistics, whose research interests cover subjects as broad as Indo-European Morphology (esp. verb), history of Indo-European Culture and Religion, onomastic; etymology, historical grammar of Greek (esp. verb), Greek dialectology and epigraphy. Professor Sowa has published widely on a range of subjects in leading peer-reviewed journals and has disseminated his research in Polish, German and English.

*****

FLORIAN STEGER has been a full professor and director of the Institute of the History, Theory and Ethics of Medicine at the University of Ulm since July 2016. Prior to this, he held the same position at the Institute of the History and Ethics of Medicine at the Martin Luther University Halle-Wittenberg from 2011. In 2018, he was awarded the 'Universitatis Lodziensis Amico' medal by the University of Łódź (Poland), and he became an honorary professor at Semmelweis University, Budapest (Hungary). He was made a corresponding member of the Saxon Academy of Sciences in 2019 and the Göttingen Academy of Sciences in 2020. In 2021, he became a full member of the Heidelberg Academy of Sciences. In 2022, the Austrian Academy of Sciences elected him a Corresponding Member Abroad.

*****

TONY WHYTON is a cultural musicologist and professor of jazz studies at Royal Birmingham Conservatoire, Birmingham City University. Whyton is the author and editor of several books including *Jazz Icons: Heroes Myths and the Jazz Tradition* (CUP, 2010) and *Beyond a Love Supreme: John Coltrane and the Legacy of an Album* (Oxford University Press 2013). As an editor, he co-founded the *Jazz Research Journal* and co-edited the *Routledge Companion to Jazz Studies* (Routledge 2018). Whyton currently co-edits the Routledge series *Transnational Studies in Jazz*. Since 2010, Whyton has led two large-scale European research projects: *Rhythm Changes: Jazz Cultures and European Identities* (HERA JRPI 2010–2013) and *Cultural Heritage and Improvised Music in European Festivals – CHIME* (JPI Cultural Heritage 2015–2018). From 2017–23, Whyton worked as a Knowledge Exchange and Impact Fellow for HERA.

Index

italic page numbers refer to an illustration; *n* refers to a note

9/11 (11th September 2001) 174, 198–99

A
Academy of Art and Design FHNW 138
Adorno, Theodor 167
African-Brazilians 182, 189–90
alcoholic drinks 118
Alexievich, Svetlana *Chernobyl Prayer* 199
algorithms 129, 132, 135, 206–07
Amsterdam 113–14
anamensis 47
Anatolia 4
Ancient Greece 94–96, 99–100
anti-mask movements 133–34, 141, 163, 164
anti-vaccine movements 164–67, 172
Aquarius (film) 184
Aristotle 49, 151
Arnuwanda II, Hittite King 4
artificial intelligence (AI) 129
Asclepius (god) 94
Atget, Eugène 199
Athens 94–96, 99–100
Atherton, Rachel *Missing/Unspecified: Demographic Data Visualization During the Covid-19 Pandemic* 135–36

B
Babette, Paul 110
Bacurau (film) *181*, 181–91
Barwick, Peter 85

Beiguelan, Giselle
 Coronario 197, (screenshot) *202*, *203*, 208
 'Coronario/Coronary' 202–03
Belarus election (2020) 55
Belcher, Kimberly 41
Benjamin, Walter 199, 200, 208
Berlin Wall, fall of (1989) 199
Black Death (1346–53) 41, 83, 98, 108–09
 images of 43
Black Lives Matter 200
Boccaccio, Giovanni *Decameron* 98, 161–62
Bodnar, Adam 63
Boghurst, William 76
Bökel, Johann 110–11, 118
Bolsonaro, Jair 184, 185–86, 202–03, 208
Boyle, Robert 118
Bradwell, Stephen 115
Brannon, Philip *The Illustrated Historical and Picturesque Guide to Corfe Castle* 20–21
Brazil 182–83, 202–03
 and slavery 189
Britain 8, 18, 22
Brooke, Humphrey 85
Brown, Allan 22
Byzantium 97, 98

C
Cairo, Alberto *How Charts Lie* 132
Callaghan, Sara 128

241

Calloway, Cab *St James Infirmary* (song) 217
    record label *214*
Camus, Albert *The Plague* 55, 101, 161, 215–22
    book jacket *214*
Can't Touch This: Covid-19 in the Contexts of Protests in Hong Kong (curated cluster) 139
Canuti, Benedictus 83
Carpenter, John 'Night' (film music) 189
Cartography of Covid-19 [Rodighiero et al.] 138
Center for Disease Control and Prevention (US) 135
Center for Systems Science and Engineering Dashboard (US) 127, 129–31
Chatterji, Sria 138
Chau, Annlin *Humanities Matter* (screenshot) *227*
Chillon, Jean-Marc 49
China 139
    assumed origin of Covid-19 pandemic 203
Christian liturgy 39, 41–50
church services 47–51, 117
    distancing in 46–49
    streaming of *38*, 46, 48, 50
civil disobedience 59
civil liberties, restrictions on 101
civil rights 64–65
coffee 119
cognitive linguistics 151, 153
Collective and Open Data Distribution-Keralam (CODD-K) 136–37, 143
collective worship 117
Conde, Miguel 186
conspiracy theories 99, 162–67
construal level theory (CLT) 29
Cooke, Jennifer 219
Corfe Castle *17*, 17–32, *25*

    impact of Covid-19 on 23–24, 26–27, 30–32
    and tourism 19–27
Council of Europe 58
Covid-19 pandemic 4, 6–9, 18–19
    government measures for 108–09
    impact on health services of 100–01
    newspaper headlines *157*, *159*
    nostalgia for a safer past 26–27
    Open Research Dataset 138
    public discourse on 158–76
    for topics related to Covid-19 *see* the topic e.g. algorithms; civil rights
    see also specific countries
Covid Denialism (curated cluster) 139
Covid E-Lit-Digital Art from the Pandemic (exhibition 2021) 195, *196*
Creighton, Charles 74, 76, 86
Critical Media Lab 138, 143
Croatia 58
Cruikshank, George *A Cart for Transporting the Dead in London* 107, *108*

D

Dadaism 200, 205
Dance of Death (image) 82
Daniel, Sharon and Erik Loyer *Exposed* 197
data curation 137–40, *140*
data visualization 129, 133–43
Day, John 77
de Chirico, Giorgio 199
Defoe, Daniel
    Due Preparations for the Plague 118
    Journal of the Plague Year 76, 108, 115–16
Dekker, Thomas 77
    Blacke Rod, The 77
    London Looke Back 77
    Meeting of Gallants, The 77
    News from Graves-End 77

Rod for Run-awayes, A 77
Seven Deadly Sins, The 77, 78
Wonderfull Yeare, The 72, 77, 78–84, 88–89
Department of Clinical Pharmacology, Mumbai 140–41
Descriptive Guide to Bournemouth, Christchurch, Wimborne and Corfe Castle 21
Development of Tourism Act (1969) 22
digital art 194–99
disease *see* illness and disease
distance *see* psychological distance; social distance; time distance
Docetism 48
Donati, Pierpaulo 49
Dong, Ensheng 129–30
Dorling, Danny 143*n*
Dornelles, Juliano 182
Durkheim, Émile 46

E
effluvia 112
electronic literature 194–95, 206–08
Electronic Literature Organization Conference (2021) 195–97
Elizabeth I, Queen, funeral of 73
ELMCIP (Electronic Literature as a Model of Creativity and Innovation) 195
England, plague in 72–75, 86–87
epidemics 4, 109, 194
   see also pandemics; Spanish flu
Erlickas, Juozas 164
Errl, Astrid 194, 197–98, 208
escapism 18–19, 30–32
EU Charter of Fundamental Rights 58
Eucharist 41–44, 49
European Convention on Human Rights and Fundamental Freedoms 58
European Court of Human Rights (ECrtHR) 58–59, 60
'Explaining the Gap: Visualizing One's Predictions Improves Recall and Comprehension of the Data' [Kim et al.] 141
eye-centrism 50

F
Fabyan, Robert *Newe Cronycles of Englande and Fraunce* 78
Facebook 133, 163, 203
Filho, Kleber Mendonça 182, 184
Finn, Ed 135
flagellants 41
Flanagan, Kieran 41
Floyd, George 55
Foucault, Michel 8–9, 128
Fracastoro, Girolamo 98
Francis, Pope 43
Frisch, Evan 174

G
Galen of Pergamum 111
game theory 46
Gaza 194
Geographic Information System 129–30
Germany *see also* Hamburg 101
Ghebreyesus, Adhanom 151
Glisson, Francis 85
Global Initiative on Psychiatry 173
gloves, in Christian liturgy 44–45
Google 197, 202, 208
Google Trends 203–04
Great Fire of London (1666) 88, 109
Grimm, Samuel Hieronymus 19
Grosser, Ben
   Endless Doomscroller, The 194, 204–05, (screenshot) 204
   USA COVID-19 deaths visualized by the footprint of the 9/11 Memorial in NYC (screenshot) 198, 208
Grzesiowski, Pawel 156

H

Hamburg 109–10, 111, 112, 113–14, 117, 118, 120*n*
Hamilton, Sir Edward Walter 20
Han, Byung-Chul *Palliativgesellschaft* (2020) 100
Harari, Juval N. *Homo Deus: A Brief History of Tomorrow* 150, 156
Hardy, Thomas *The Hand of Ethelberta* 21
Harvey, Gideon 114
Harwood, Robert W. *I Went Down to St James Infirmary* 218
Hayles, N. Katherine 207
Henslowe, Philip 77
Heritage After Lockdown project 28
Herring, Francis 115
heterotopia 49–50
Hippocrates 94
Hippocratic Corpus 94, 96
Hirsch, Silvia *Confluence of Institutional Violence and Structural Poverty in Low-Income Neighbourhoods of Argentina* 139
Hittite cuneiform tablets 3, 5–6
Hittite Empire 4–5
HIV/AIDS 194
Hodges, Nathaniel 77–78
    Loimologia, or an Historical Account of the Plague in London in 1665, 71, 72, 75, 78, 84–89
Homer *Iliad* 94, 102
Homily of Toledo 43–44
Hullman, Jessica 141
human rights 57–65, 231
humanities 7, 10, 221–22, 228–32
Humanities in the European Research Area (HERA) 10, 232
humours 96–97, 111–12
Hungary 101
Huxley, Aldous 172
hygiene, ritualization of 50

I

Ibn Al-Khatib 83–84
Ibn Khatima 83
illness and disease 7–8
    as a metaphor 7–9
    theurgic models of 94, 97
Institute of Experimental Design and Media 138
International Covenant on Civil and Political Rights 57
intoxicants 117–18
Israel and Gaza 194
Istanbul Convention 166, 167

J

Jacob (patriarch) 44
Jacobi, Johannes *De Pestilencia* 83
Jagiellonian University, Institute of Journalism 153
Jakučiunas, Andrius 163, 166
Jedinstva (pro-Soviet organisation) 169, 170
Jews, accused of causing plague 99
John VI Cantacuzenus, Emperor of Byzantium 98, 104
Johns Hopkins University 129, 130, 131–32, 135, 143
Johnson, Boris 8
Jokūbaitis, Alvydas 168
Jones, Colin 110
Jonson, Ben 77
Jurkevičius, Paulius 167
Justinian Plague (from 541 ADE) 97

K

Kaye, Sir Richard 19
Kephale, Richard 115

Knight of Light Pierces the Dragon of Darkness with his Spear of Reason (game) 163
Kracauer, Siegfried 202, 208

L
Lagoeiro, Carlos 189
Lakoff, George *Women, Fire and Dangerous Things* 152
Lakoff, George and Evan Frisch 174
Landsbergis, Vytautas 170, 171
language 151–57, 175–76
    and conceptualizing (cartoon) *149*
    impact of pandemics on 151, 171–75, 202–03, 207
    naming of difficult words (cartoon) *154*
    see also Lithuanian language; Portuguese language
late internet 132–33
Lazarus (Biblical parable) 82
Lee, Sir Robert 72
Legare, Cristine 41
Lima, Mauricio 199
literary allegory 166–67
literature 228
Lithuania 158–76
    commemoration of 1918 Independence (2022) 170
Lithuanian Family Movement March (2021) 166, 167, 168
Lithuanian language
    change in meaning of words 171–75
    A Wordle of Coronavirus 160
Lloyd, A.L. 218
Lodge, Thomas *A Treatise of the Plague* (1603) 83
London plague 72–89, 108–09
    chemists 86
    City of London 73–5, 78–79
    doctors 83, 85–86
    government measures for 87–89, 108, 114–15
    herbal remedies for 80
    mortality rates 73–77, 86–87, 109
    nurses 85–86
    Reflections on the Weekly Bills of Mortality 74
Long, Paul 217
Loukissas, Yanni Alexander *All Data are Local* 135, 137–38
Lowenthal, David 18, 27, 31
Loyer, Erik 197
Lydgate, John *The Fall of Princes* 82
Lynteris, Christos 209

M
Marlowe, Christopher *The Great Tamburlaine* 80
Marston, John 77
masks 56, 98, 120, 130, 203
    in Christian liturgy 45 *see also* anti-mask movement
Massachussetts Institute of Technology (MIT) 133
Massey, Doreen 190
Massinger, Philip 77
Mattos, R. 188
Mažeikis, Gintautas 162, 163–64, 167
Mbembe, Achille 182
McConchie, Alan 131–32, 142–43
    Visualizing the Pulse of a Pandemic (blog) 142
memory
    collective memory 198, 218, 231
    public memory 199, 228
    ritual memory 40
mental illness 101
miasma 110–11, 114, 120
military metaphors 174

Ministry of Housing and Local Government (UK) 22
Mohammed, Bilal *Lost Inside: A Digital Inquiry* 197
Montagne, Véronique 84
Morton, Timothy 199, 208
Munganga (theatre group) 189
Mursilis II, Hittite King 4–5, 228

N
Napiórkowski, Marcin 150
National Heritage List for England 22
National Preventive Mechanism 61
National Trust 23
Neighbouring Sounds (film) 184
Netherlands, assumed origin of Plague 72, 75
New York Times 131, 143
night and nocturnal time-space 182, 184–85, 189–90
Norway: Black Death in (1349–50) 13*n*

O
Office for Democratic Institutions and Human Rights (ODIHR) 59
Orwell, George 172–73
  Politics and the English Language 175

P
Paget, Nathan 85
pandemics 9, 128, 194
  and liminality 49
Passover ritual 40
Paul, Saint 48
Pawłowska, Danuta 'Coronavirus in the World' 155
pax (ritual plates) 46
Peloponnesian War (431–404 BC) 94–95
Pepys, Samuel 115, 119
Pereira, Silvero 186–87
Perera, Jamie *Sonification of UK Covid Deaths* 139
Pickstock, Catherine 47–48
Pie Tavern, London 116
Piringer, Jorg
  Covid-19 genome (sound poem) 206–07
  'Quarantine TV' (screenshot) *193*
Places of Joy survey 19, 24
plague hospitals 113
Plague Orders (1603) 73, 79, 88, 115
Plague Prayers 4–6, 9, 117, 228
plagues 94
  assumed origins of 80, 86, 98, 99, 110–11
  bubonic and pneumonic plague 110
  marking houses with crosses 87, 108, 114–15, 119
  medical writings on 83–84
  as a metaphor 6, 7–9, 110
  psychological interpretations of 7–8
  as punishment by God 5, 43, 84, 97, 112
  Second Plague Pandemic 108–09
  therapies for 96–97
  transmission of 111, 120 *see also* epidemics; Black Death; Covid-19; Justinian Plague; pandemics; SARS and specific countries
Poland 55–65, 101, 151, 155, 231
  protest against abortion laws 54, 60–64
  and reform of judiciary 59–61
  Women's Strike 60
  'Wujek' coal mine protest movement (1981) 56
Polish Catholicism 43
Polish Constitutional Tribunal (CT) 57, 60, 61, 62
poor people 75, 81–82, 88–89, 113, 116, 186 *see also* rich people

Portuguese language 182, 189, 203
Princeton Center for Digital Humanities 138
Procopius of Caesarea *De Bello Persico* 97, 98, 103–04
protest movements 55–56
Przyłębska, Julia 59–60, 61–62, 63, 64
psychological distance 29–31
public houses 114–16
public spaces, cleaning of 113–14
purse nets 83
Putin, Vladimir 231

Q
QR codes 173
quarantine 8, 98, 109, 113 *see also* specific countries

R
Rachlevičius, Vidas 168–69, 170
religious rituals 39
rich people 75, 81–83, 84, 88–89, 148
    see also poor people
right to assembly 56–59
Rincon, Gomez 42
rituals 39–51
Rousseff, Dilma 184, 186
Royal College of Physicians 73, 78, 88–89, 115
Rubinstein, B. 187
Russia
    invasion of Ukraine by 194, 209, 221, 230–31
    political protests in 58
Ryall's New Weymouth Guide (1790) 19–20

S
Sadauskas-Kvietkevičius, Romas 167
Sadurski, Wojciech 59
St James Infirmary (song) 216–19
St John's Cathedral, Toruń 43

Sample, Mark
    Content Moderator Sim (game) 205–06
    Infinite Catalog of Crushed Dreams, The 197, 206, 207–09
Sariola, Salla *Necropolitics of Vaccine Capitalism* 138–39
SARS-Cov-2 virus 4, 151, 194
Sartre, Jean-Paul *Nausea* 217
satire 116–17
science, attitudes to 166–67, 171–72
senses 112
Silva, Lula Ignaçio da 186
Simpson, William *Zenexton Anti-Pestilentiale* (1665) 118
Singh, Julietta 209
Siu, Margaret *Covid-19 Propaganda in China* 139
Skarga, Barbara *Identity and Difference* 153
Slack, Paul 74–75, 77, 83
smell 112, 113
social contact 114–15
social distance 29–30, 45–46, 100–01, 108, 173
social isolation 110–11
Social Distancing (journal) 159
SocietyNow#1 competition 153
Sontag, Susan *Illness as Metaphor* 7–8, 154
Spanish flu epidemic (1918–19) 194, 197–98
Stockholm 114
Stow, John 72
    Annales 74
    Survay of London 82
sugar 118–19
Suppiluliuma I, Hittite Emperor 4

T
Taussig, Michael 199–200, 205, 208
tea 119
technology, and pandemics 128–43
tele-liturgy *see* church services

Thomism 41, 44
Thucydides *History of the Peloponnesian War* 94–95, 98, 99, 102–03
Tienanmen Square protest movement (1989) 56
time distance, in Christian liturgy 47
tobacco 118–19
Town and Country Planning Acts (1944, 1947) 22
Triumph of Death (fresco 1446) 93
Tropicalia movement, Brazil 187–88
Trump, Donald 203
tularemia (rabbit fever) 4
Turner, Victor 49
Twitter 132, 133
Tzara, Tristan 205

U
Ukraine, Russian invasion of 194, 209, 221, 230–31
UN Human Rights Committee 57
United States 43, 55, 131–32, 135, 167, 196, 199

V
vaccine passports 164–65, 167, 171
vaccines 9, 95, 156, 164, 167–68 *see also* anti-vaccine movement
Valatka, Rimvydas 164–65, 167
Valleriole, François *Traicté de la Peste* 83
Vasiliauskaité, Nida 163, 164, 166–67
Vėgėlė, Ignas 168
Veloso, Caetano *Objeto não Identificado* (song) 187–88
Venice Commission 59
Viral Visualization: How Coronovirus Skeptics Use Orthodox Data Practices to Promote Unorthodox Science Online (MIT) 133, 134
Visualizing Covid-19 as a Zoonotic Disease 139
Visualizing the Virus (platform) 138–40

W
war metaphor 174
Washington Post 131
Weiser, Peg Brand 220
Welte, Bernhard 40
Weymouth and Melcome Regis New Guide (1835) 20
Weymouth Guide (1785) 19
Wharton, Thomas 85
White Privilege and Covid-19 (curated cluster) 139
Williams, Robert 182, 190
World Health Organization 56, 151

Y
Yersin, Alexandre 98
yersinias pestis (plague) 4, 98, 120

Z
Zellen, Jody
    Avenue S Ghost City 200–02
    screenshot *201*